PROGRESS IN COMMUNITY CHILD HEALTH
Volume One

Edited by

NICK SPENCER MPhil, FRCP, DCH
Professor of Community Child Health,
School of Postgraduate Medical Education,
University of Warwick, Coventry, UK

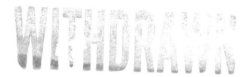

CHURCHILL LIVINGSTONE
EDINBURGH HONG KONG LONDON MADRID MELBOURNE NEW YORK AND
TOKYO 1995

CHURCHILL LIVINGSTONE
Medical Division of Pearson Professional Limited

Distributed in the United States of America by Churchill
Livingstone Inc., 650 Avenue of the Americas, New York,
N.Y. 10011, and by associated companies, branches and
representatives throughout the world.

© Pearson Professional Limited 1995

First published 1995

ISBN 0 443 051976
ISSN 1 357 7675

British Library Cataloguing in Publication Data
A catalogue record for this book is available from the British Library

Library of Congress Cataloguing in Publication Data is available

Produced by Longman Singapore Publishers (Pte) Ltd.
Printed in Singapore

PROGRESS IN
COMMUNITY
CHILD HEALTH

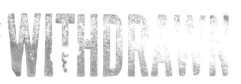

Don Gresswell Ltd., London, N.21   Cat. No. 1208   DG 02242/71

PROGRESS IN COMMUNITY CHILD HEALTH

Provisional Contents of Volume 2
Edited by Nick Spencer

Contents

Preface

This is the first of a new annual series aimed at community child health professionals, particularly community paediatricians and community child health nurses. It inherits the mantle of the series edited by Aidan Macfarlane *Progress in Child Health*; hopefully, it will be possible to maintain the high standards set by Aidan's highly acclaimed series. 'Community' has been added to the series title to emphasise the focus on community-based approaches to child health.

The series has two main objectives: firstly, to provide a much needed theoretical backdrop to the work of community child health professionals and secondly, to offer up-to-date key points for clinical practice related to commonly encountered aspects of community-based child health care. It has a primarily UK focus but as can be seen from this volume, the editorial net has been (and will be, in the future) thrown beyond these shores in search of the most authoritative contributors.

In thinking about this series, I have considered the component elements of community child health and community paediatrics as practised in the UK. Community paediatrics has developed from a number of separate strands; developmental paediatrics, child health surveillance and screening, epidemiology and 'population paediatrics', educational and school medicine, behavioural paediatrics and social paediatrics (in the UK, principally concerned with child protection and 'looked after' children). A relative newcomer but increasing in importance is ambulatory paediatrics–an American term, referring, in the UK community paediatic context, to the delivery of paediatric care to children with non-urgent paediatric problems in settings outside the hospital ward and incorporates primary care paediatrics and the primary–secondary care interface. Given these different and, often disparate, elements, UK community paediatricians can be excused for wondering what major area of responsibility they are going to be asked to undertake next.

The subject areas chosen for the series chapters broadly follow these component elements of community child health. In addition, they are chosen to reflect the multi-disciplinary and multi-agency nature of community child health work and include authors from allied disciplines. In recognition of the management and decision-making role of many community child health professionals, authors have been asked, where appropriate, to incorporate advice for medical and nursing managers into their chapters and some chapters specifically addressing purchaser/provider issues have been commissioned.

The first and last chapters of this first volume are written by Lennart Köhler and Michel Manciaux respectively, two of the most distinguished European and international social paediatricians. Professor Köhler argues the need for a 'new child public health' as a counterbalance to superspecialised and fragmented paediatrics. Professor Manciaux, in his impassioned statement of the health care needs of poor families and their children, shows exactly why the 'new child public health' approach with its emphasis on placing the health of children in its full social, economic and political context is essential in meeting the needs of the poorest and most vulnerable in our societies.

Tony Waterston addresses a similar theme from the standpoint of child health services demonstrating tested practical contributions which they can make to the reduction of child health inequalities. Lip-service is paid to equity in service delivery in the new look health service: Dr Waterston's chapter offers providers and purchasers properly evaluated interventions to turn talk into action.

One of the apparent recent successes of a national health promotion campaign has been the 'Back-to Sleep' campaign aimed at reducing the incidence of sudden infant deaths. Ruth Gilbert examines the background to the campaign and assesses its success concluding that parents have responded by putting their children to sleep on their backs with a resultant fall in the incidence of unexpected deaths. Dr Gilbert points out that the likelihood of finding an explanation for death in infants who die suddenly and unexpectedly has increased as the incidence of SIDS has fallen, re-emphasising the need for thorough investigation of each infant death.

Hearing screening is amongst the most widely researched community-based screening procedures in infancy. In recent years, the health visitor 8-month hearing screen has been subjected to detailed scrutiny, some areas have abandoned their screening programmes in favour of 'at risk' neonatal screening and increasing parental awareness. Adrian Davis explores the background to the controversy and makes some clear recommendations to those setting up or reviewing hearing screening programmes.

Parental participation and partnership with parents have become 'buzz words' amongst child care professionals. These often misinterpreted and misused concepts are explored by Peter Appleton with particular reference to child development centres. He highlights the benefits to the child and family and the probable long-term resource saving of a healthy parent-professional relationship whilst stressing that 'good practice' in this area is not easy and is time-consuming requiring skilled listening and sensitive information-giving. Again there are important lessons here for both providers of child development services and purchasers.

Gabrielle Laing reviews the evidence for effectiveness and efficiency of preschool vision screening, next to hearing screening the most widely practised preschool screening programme. She points out that the natural history of normal and abnormal visual development remains poorly understood making it difficult to design a rational vision screening programme. Amblyopia, the main rationale for early vision screening, remains ill-understood and there is doubt as to whether early treatment results in long-term improvement. If preschool screening for visual defects is to be continued, Dr Laing stresses that its effectiveness and efficiency should be regularly monitored.

The prevalence of behaviour problems in preschool children seems to be increasing. They form a major part of the workload of all child health professionals whether community or hospital based. Paul Stallard presents imaginative approaches to the problem which recognise the key importance of parental definition of the problem and make positive use of parental skills. He proposes that assessment of preschool behaviour should become an integral part of child health surveillance and suggests a simple questionnaire which has been used effectively in Bath.

Current issues in educational medicine are covered in Chapters 8 and 9; Tricia David, an educationalist specialising in early childhood education, explores the education/health interface in early childhood development and Mike Bannon looks at the increasing problem of the role of teachers in the relation to children with chronic illness.

Professor David concludes with a timely warning that if we create a society which leaves the provision of services to very young children to market forces we must recognise that there will be long-term costs. She stresses the important role of education and health services as advocates for young children. Dr Bannon reviews the literature related to teachers' awareness and knowledge of chronic childhood illness and addresses the thorny problem of the 'in loco parentis' role. He suggests strategies both national and local for clarifying the teachers role, increasing teachers' awareness, improving health service communication with teachers and providing support to teachers in the increasingly stressful role of dealing with chronic childhood illness in the school setting.

John James, himself a GP in a deprived inner-city area, considers the delivery of comprehensive child care services in primary care. Dr James explores the implications of increased GP responsibility for child health services highlighting the opportunities which primary care offers in the development of comprehensive child health care services in particular the development and implementation of a philosophy of child care based on the principle of equity, close teamwork with community paediatricians and improved collection and use of relevant data to determine the allocation of resources and to provide a tool for advocacy.

'Looked after' children are amongst the most vulnerable, have the greatest needs and are frequently the most neglected by the child health services. Dr Buck and colleagues present a strong argument for changing this situation and illustrate how community child health services can be geared to the needs of these children using imaginative approaches such as the 'health passport', a health record held by the child which is in direct line of descent from the parent-held record. Continuity of care, whenever possible, comprehensive and sensitive assessment and high levels of collaboration between health and social services are seen as essential first steps in the provision of a high quality of service to these children.

To show that this series also adheres to the principle of continuity, Chapter 12 is written by Aidan Macfarlane who has now moved to the exalted status of child and adolescent health commissioner. Dr Macfarlane is an acknowledged expert on adolescent medicine and here he addresses the commissioning of health services for adolescents. He deals with a range of services for adolescents stressing throughout the importance of empowering adolescents and giving them control over their own lives and the services offered to them. His chapter will be of particular interest to those who are struggling with the problems of achieving 'Health of the Nation' targets in relation to adolescents. He echoes the message which comes across in many of the chapters — health is a social and political phenomenon, not just a biological state and it is influenced as much by social and political policies as by health services provision.

It is a particular honour and pleasure for me to be asked to 'pick up' the threads sewn so competently by Aidan Macfariane in the original *Progress in child health* series. I hope that the readers will get as much from this varied collection of chapters as I have, they will not all suit every taste but I hope that all community child health professionals will find something here of interest to them and of relevance to their work.

Coventry   N.J.S.
1995

Contributors

Peter Appleton PhD
Clinical Psychology Services Manager and Honorary Lecturer in Clinical Psychology, Department of Paediatrics, Wrexham Maelor Hospital, Wrexham, Clwyd, UK

Michael J. Bannon MB, MA, DCH, MSc(IT), FRCP(I)
Consultant Paediatrician and Honorary Senior Clinical Lecturer, Cape Road Clinic, Warwick, UK

Sandra Buck MB, ChB, DCH
Member of the Institute of Psycosexual Medicine, Meadows Health Centre, The Meadows, Nottingham, UK

Tricia David BSc, MA
Senior Lecturer in Education, Institute of Education, Warwick University, Coventry, UK

Adrian Davis PhD, MSc
Head of the Department of Epidemiology and Public Health, MRC Institute of Hearing Research, University of Nottingham, Nottingham, UK

François-Paul Debionne MD
International Movement ATD Fourth World, Strasbourg, France

Caroline de Cates BSc, MB BS, MRCP, MSc
Northwest Anglia Healthcare Trust, Horsefair Clinic, Wisbeach, Cambridgeshire, UK

Ruth Gilbert MD, MRCP, MB ChB, MSc
Lecturer in Epidemiology, Department of Epidemiology and Biostatistics, Institute of Child Health, London, UK

John James MB ChB, MRCGP
General Practitioner, Montpellier Health Centre, Bristol, UK

Lennart Köhler MD, PhD
Professor of Social Paediatrics and Dean, Nordic School of Public Health, Göteborg, Sweden

Gabrielle Laing MSc, MRCP, DCH
Senior Registrar in Community Child Health, South Western Hospital,
Stockwell, London, UK

J. Aiden MacFarlane MB, BChir, MA, FRCP
Consultant Community Paediatrician, Department of Public Health
Medicine, Headington, Oxford, UK

Michel R. G Manciaux MD, FRCP
Professor (Emeritus) of Public Health, University of Nancy, Nancy, France

Y. K. Ng BSc, MB BS, MRCP, DRCOG, DCH
Consultant Community Paediatrician, Nottingham Community Health
NHS Trust, Nottingham, UK

Leon Polnay
University Hospital, Nottingham, UK

Paul Stallard BSc, MSc, CPsycol, AFBPsS
Child and Adolscent Psychology Manager, Psychology Department,
Department of Child and Family Psychiatry, Royal United Hosptital, Bath,
UK

Tony Waterson
Consultant Paediatrician, Newcastle General Hospital,
Newcastle-upon-Tyne, UK

1. New child public health

L. Köhler

MEDICINE AND HEALTH

Most professionals involved in community child health services have a clinical background and thereby a formal training that has concentrated on tracing, caring and alleviating diseases, disorders and deviations in children and young people. This is a task that demands knowledge, skills, empathy and understanding of the individual child, his development and environment.

Children's health, however, is a much broader and positive concept, addressing many more aspects of children's well-being than their medical care. Many atttempts have been made to define health, and however they differ there is a general agreement that it is a positive and multidimensional state; it is not only freedom from disease that is at stake. Most well-known and still most quoted is the definition of health given in the 1946 constitution of the World Health Organization (WHO): 'a state of complete physical, mental and social well-being and not merely the absence of disease or infirmity'. Although this definition has been heavily criticized, on the grounds that it is imprecise, utopian and impractical, it has undeniably made its impact on the debate on health. It should therefore be noted that it does stress the positive nature of health, and in its notion of well-being it expands the concept beyond physical health or fitness.

Today, many prefer a concept of health that is connected to the individual's situation and allows them to cope with the demands of life. Thereby, health is the ability to resist endurance of a physical, mental and social nature, so that it does not lead to reduced lifespan, function or well-being. These thoughts have been more poetically expressed by the Danish author and scientist Piet Hein:

Health is not bought with a chemist's pills,
nor saved by the surgeon's knife.
Health is not only the absence of ills,
but the fight for the fullness of life.

The WHO concept of health was to some extent clarified in 1977 when the World Health Assembly adopted the resolution known as 'Health for all by the year 2000'.[1] This stated, as a central objective of member states' social policy goals, a level of health to enable everyone to achieve a socially and economically productive life. Thus, health is a resource for everyday life, not the objective of living. The underlying philosophy or ideology of this goal is equity: equity within and between countries, and social justice in health. But the goal became more than ideology when it was developed into a strategy with 38 targets for Europe, accepted by all the member states.[2] In 1991 the targets were updated and a new target on ethics was added.[3] They now represent a common European view of what could and should be done to achieve health for all. These targets place emphasis on promotion of healthier lifestyles and a healthy environment and on the reorientation of health care towards a broad concept of community-based primary health care.

PUBLIC HEALTH

In the traditional education and training of health personnel, there is little to be found of topics that are important in this connection, i.e. community health, epidemiology, environmental health, health education, leadership, health economics. An educational programme with such a broad and comprehensive view must be built on a multidisciplinary approach, based on social, humanistic, natural and, of course, medical sciences; thus we are in fact describing public health science — a multidisciplinary area with special reference to the influence of social structure, environment and care system on the health of the population. Or, as it is defined in Sir Donald Acheson's influential report on public health in England: 'Public health is the science and art of preventing disease, prolonging life and promoting health through organised efforts of society'.[4]

This report also introduced the concept of the 'new public health' or, as it was later designated, the 'renaissance of public health'. The 'old public health' was concentrating on the 'sanitary idea' where health hazards were drained away, burned or buried. The limitations of that framework of thinking about public health have been increasingly exposed in the growth of ecological knowledge and awareness, a new consciousness of the finite resources of the planet and of each generation's responsibility for their stewardship — a realization that man exists in nature not above or outside it. These are among the essential planks in the 'new public health' platform. The 'new public health' thus deals with maximizing public involvement in health, and with making promotion of better health a responsibility of decision-makers in all organizations in all sectors of the economy — manufacturing and services, public and private.[5]

CHILD HEALTH

Action on these issues in order to enhance population health is referred to as the public health function. Naturally, this includes the whole population, but there are several major reasons why children's health and well-being is of special importance in public health:

1. Children make up a substantial part of the country's population — in Europe generally around 20%.
2. Children represent a vulnerable group in society, and their health and well-being thus reflect the will and ability of the society to care for its citizens.
3. Children have no political power and are not represented in formal or informal pressure groups able to influence health and related policies.
4. The foundations of adult health as well as knowledge, attitudes and behaviour in health matters are learned and laid in the formative years of childhood and youth.
5. The United Nations have proposed special protection for children through their Convention of Rights of the Child, adopted in 1989.

WHO had already in its constitution identified 'the basic importance' of the 'healthy development of the child' and 'the (child's) ability to live harmoniously in a changing total environment'. The European 'health for all strategy' made the explicit claim that what is at stake in the achievement of the targets is nothing less than the future of the children of Europe. A special and very strong emphasis in this strategy is put on the concept of health promotion.

Health protection and promotion as a child health issue

The concepts of health protection and promotion have increasingly been seen as a central feature of the 'health for all strategy' as well as in public health science. The whole concept of a welfare society providing a safety network of income and other forms of support to protect its weaker or disadvantaged members should be seen as a set of health protection measures no less than traditional environment health protection or, say, classical accident prevention measures. The further role of the welfare society is to ensure that people do not, through force of circumstances, become disadvantaged but that they retain their personal resources of resilience and self-reliance which help maintain health.

Health promotion, the complementary component to protection, covers measures which are intended to support and sustain people's healthy patterns of living and to facilitate health-improving behavioural change (reducing health-risk behaviour, adopting health-enhancing behaviour), and to secure needed environmental changes which would reduce, or better eliminate, social and other environmental causes of ill-health. This basically means the process of enabling people to increase control over, and to improve, their health. This process involves the population as a whole, not only the so-called risk populations, with their particular biological and behavioural characteristics or persistent exposure to unacceptable hazards to health, and is directed towards determinants and causes of health. Action to promote population health requires the close cooperation of many sectors in society, reflecting the diversity of conditions and factors which influence health: not only legistation but also communication and education; not only organization of services but also community development and spontaneous local activities against health hazards.

The Ottawa Conference on Health Promotion 1986, cosponsored by the WHO, was the first formal occasion when the potential of promotion was fully articulated.[6] The Ottawa Charter identified the requirements of a concerted effort from different professions and others in many sectors. In terms of action areas to which that concerted effort should be directed, the Ottawa Charter identified the following as the field of concern:

- Building health promotive public policy, i.e. in all sectors and levels of society, aimed at influencing public and private decision-makers, and spanning the physical, economic, social and cultural environment.
- Creating supportive environments, i.e. in both their physical and social dimensions in settings of everyday life (work, leisure, family, etc.), strengthening the community's social support systems.
- Strengthening community action, i.e. whether community is defined by locality or as people with shared interests and objectives, people involved in debate decision and action for promoting health, drawing on people's own resources and giving them a greater sense of self-worth.
- Developing personal skills, i.e. to increase self-esteem, to strengthen people's capacities to make their own choices and to cope with the pressures they face.
- Reorienting health services, i.e. to give greater emphasis to promotion in the remit of these services and their staffs and to stress the potential of health care institutions as health promotion settings.

It should also be noted that effective health education is a necessary condition for purposeful action in health protection and promotion — both to enhance health knowledge and awareness in the population and to help create the conditions which make health supportive change possible. Health education as now understood seeks to empower people so that, individually, by making informed choices, they may adopt healthy patterns of living and, collectively, as responsible and aware citizens, they intensify political and social action for policy and structural changes as envisaged in the Ottawa Charter. It is therefore essential that the concept of health education finds a place in the mainstream of the school curriculum rather than at the margin.

The range of actions taken within a public health strategy which has the needs of children in mind and adheres to the goals and aims of health for all would need to:

- Provide education and later work in conformity with a person's physical and mental capacity.
- Raise people's awareness about health matters; enable them to cope with health problems by helping them develop personal skills; provide them

with valid information on such basic matters of lifestyle as appropriate diet, physical activity, relaxation and sleep.
• Strengthen support to community efforts of self-care and self-reliance through the steady availability of professional advice and services where needed, to ensure that community action develops and is sustained in a way which most effectively protects and promotes the community's health.

Basic to this new look at health, centred around protection, prevention and especially promotion, is the concept of 'empowerment' — the realization that health cannot be reached without the active involvement and actual responsibility of people themselves. There is no such thing as a total professional taking over of a responsibility — the patients or the clients should always be involved. In these sentences it is not difficult to recognize the line of thinking that has gone into the whole public sector during the last decade or so, most obvious perhaps within the health and social services: the professionals can advise but decisions on their lives should be taken by individuals.

There is a good illustration of the historical development of the official view of the role of professionals towards target groups to be seen in the overall objectives of the child health services in Sweden (Table 1.1); from a purely bureaucratic, professional statement, to a supportive and activating approach, to coming close to a partnership as propounded in the last statement, which is, however, not yet official.

CHILD PUBLIC HEALTH

Thus, the ideologies of 'health for all', public health and children's health merge in 'social paediatrics' or, as we may call it, 'child public health', the tasks of which are to place the health of children and their families in their full social, economic and political context. In our times of superspecialization and fragmentation of medical sciences and medical professions, so obvious in clinical paediatrics, child public health is the counterbalance, with its intersectoral and multidisciplinary approach to the fullness of health.

Table 1.1   Objectives of child health services in Sweden

1969
A complete health surveillance and a handicap finding activity

1979
Support and activate the parents in their parenthood and thereby create favourable conditions for a comprehensive development of children

1995
To promote the health of children and their families by enabling them to take responsibility for their own self-development

Child public health thus implies a very broad concept, taking professionals away from the narrow experience of the specialized institutions into the community, making them aware of the social context in which children live in order to better understand their health problems, and also the need to promote genuine interdisciplinary and interprofessional team working. Thus, it means that the clinical practice of physicians, the caring tasks of nurses and others, and the work of child public health will be seen as complementary and not as entities competing for professional esteem, public recognition, and political and financial support.

Child public health as a field of study and action has three principal concerns.[5] First, it is concerned with the education, training and career development of child health workers. Secondly, there is research in its various forms, conducted on a multi- and interdisciplinary basis, designed to increase understanding of different child health phenomena and to clarify the desirability and feasibility of policy measures and programmes to improve children's health. Thirdly, there is service provision, working with practitioners on policies and problems and also accepting responsibility for ensuring that a participating community is an informed community, whether it be political representatives, community action groups, voluntary health workers of various kinds or the professional workers in other sectors where actions have a potential impact on children's health.

In education it is important to instill public health values and perspectives in a consistent and continuing way to practitioners and academics, from undergraduate through postgraduate to postexperience education.

The second task is that of research. A conventional argument has it that research work keeps the educator intellectually sharp and enriches the teaching. The teacher who is active in research is a better teacher. This is probably true, but the duty of research is also to determine how matters are interconnected. It is vital that public health research relates to the world, is practical and relevant, and it might be that the research developed in this way will adopt a somewhat different set of underlying values than those of the classical elitist academic world. Of course this does not mean abandoning a certain sense of detachment in analysing problems, the ability to see more than one side to a problem, the ability to think through the implications and consequences of alternative courses of action or the search for truth. But public health cannot confine itself only to those activities that follow the rules of academic science. In the real world actions have sometimes to be taken on assumptions and judgement, showing empathy with fellow health workers doing a practical job, and indeed with colleagues in all other sectors working for children's health.

Thirdly, there is the task of service. The same considerations apply as for research, that child public health become involved in ways which are seen by others to be relevant. Indeed, active involvement in service, including consulting, is arguably the best way to strengthen one's credibility as an educator with students. It can show them that academics do know the world the students are entering, that their understanding and messages to them are relevant, and that academics will be a continuing support to them in their working career. The key word, again, is relevance. The goal of a unit of child public health — whether in a university, school of public health or in a community health department — should be to demonstrate itself as a centre of relevance rather than a centre of excellence as expected in traditional academic circles. Only by leaving the ivory tower is it possible to understand the problems, to be visible and credible and to receive recognition from the public and from politicians. If we insist on equating public health with medicine we will always remain on the periphery of medicine when we could instead be at the centre of health.

Some research outcomes

From recent research programmes on children's health in general and on handicapped children in particular, some interesting observations have been made. Although the studies were performed in countries that belong to the richest in the world and, consequently, with children that are among the most healthy in the world, there are some lessons and experiences that are universal and could lead to conclusions that are generally applicable in research and education as well as in practice.[7,8]

- Children are very seldom in focus in population-based studies on health, well-being and quality of life. Consequently, the otherwise so overwhelming collection of health data does not offer a children's perspective.
- Even when children's health is seen from a public health perspective, children are regarded as a group, whose importance mainly lies in the fact that they will eventually grow up into adulthood, rather than as human beings each with their individual integrity to be respected.
- There is very little discussion about whether the traditional so-called health indicators used for adults (e.g. life expectancy and use of health services) are the most suitable for children.
- Studies of children's health are usually limited to small areas or age groups, and are only by exception representative of major areas or a country.
- Definitions of diseases and their seriousness, traditions of care and services are seldom uniform and unambiguous, and that goes for age limits, social class, geographical areas, etc. This makes the results difficult to interpret and comparisons more or less impossible.
- Too few data on children's health are based on repeated studies or follow-ups.
- Data on children's social background and living conditions are seldom encountered, either in official statistics or in research reports.

The overall conclusion, from a methodological point of view, is that there is no systematic, continuous and comprehensive reporting of children's health, seen from children's perspective and put into a social context. One recommendation, therefore, in this study was the creation of a national system to coordinate the documentation of children's health and well-being and to develop theories and methodologies. This all adds up to a strong child health research activity, which should be interdisciplinary and interprofessional, and is relevant to the needs of children, families and society.

IMPLICATIONS: AN ELEMENT OF A STRATEGY

Child public health — research as well as training and practical work — should be based on the 'health for all strategy', and place the health of children in its full social, economic and political context. It means that activities should be practical and relevant and carried out by interdisciplinary and multiprofessional teams, absorbing the insight that we have from different social sciences such as sociology, psychology, economics, organizational behaviour, political science and what can be offered by management sciences such as operational research, systems analysis, computer sciences.

With such a breadth of competence, public health is fit to confront a wide range of child health issues, be it a healthy public policy for children, social support for vulnerable groups, product safety, traffic planning or immunization uptake.

One important area to be covered by child public health is the development of health indicators that are appropriate for use among children. Vulnerable groups should be more closely observed and followed, e.g. children with chronic disease, abused children, refugees, immigrants and other underprivileged groups.

An ideal, although a seemingly idealistic and utopian, outcome of this public health research would be the development of a complete, systematic and continuous surveillance of children's health and well-being, seen from a child's perspective and placed in a social context. This would create an instrument to judge children's health, to compare it within and between countries and between periods of time, and to allow evaluation of health-promoting and disease-preventing activities in the child population.[9,10]

To take child public health to the centre of child health and keep it there, a strategy is needed. This strategy, with elements of ideology and vision as well as something still of orthodox planning, must take into account that the public sector, in all Europe, will be more deregulated, consumer- and market-oriented and outcome-responsible than has traditionally been expected of it. This implies that some methods and means, better known and used more in business life than in the public sector, might need to be employed to obtain the goals. Key elements in the strategy indicated, however, should not be very different from those traditionally followed in the best public health sector practice.

It seems evident that the first task of each public health team or unit must be to establish, or perhaps in some cases to renew, its own sense of coherence, affirming its commitment to interprofessional and interdisciplinary working and finding a focus for its efforts which harnesses the energies and interest of all the staff, i.e. the development of a strong 'corporate image'.

Secondly, there must be a conscious attempt to find allies and partners for action at all levels — local, national and international — in the professional and political spheres, paying particular attention to establishing a good relationship with the media, and finding ways of making contacts with the public at large, especially not forgetting the children themselves.

Lastly, in bodies such as ESSOP (the European Society for Social Pediatrics), ASPHER (Association of Schools of Public Health in the European Region) and EUPHA (European Public Health Association), there are means for collective action and for mutual aid and support. It is, however, a slow process to make active and powerful international forces out of professional associations, especially if most of the work has to be done by voluntary and unpaid staff.

Thus, it is evident that the issues of concern for child public health distinguish it clearly from the biomedical interests that dominate clinical paediatrics. Child public health is an open multiprofessional field whose concerns relate to child health. Clinical paediatrics as a closed medical speciality has a no less necessary but equally very different orientation to child morbidity. Most paediatricians still identify themselves more easily with clinical paediatrics, which is a well established and respected discipline in medicine, rather than with the emergent and still fluid territory of child health. It is important for those working in child public health, especially physicians, to accept that they will always be seen by fellow physicians as on the periphery of medicine. Public health workers must therefore see themselves quite clearly and unequivocally as at the centre of child health and to vigorously pursue their tasks in that spirit.

KEY POINTS FOR CLINICAL PRACTICE

- Child health is different from paediatrics, by addressing broader and more positive aspects of children's well-being than their medical care.
- An educational programme with this broad and comprehensive view should be built on a multidisciplinary approach, based on social, humanistic, natural and medical sciences.
- These aspects meet in child public health, where health promotion is a central issue, i.e. the process of enabling children and families to increase control over, and to improve, their health.
- Child public health is a counterbalance to the superspecialized and fragmented paediatrics and is, as a field of study and action, concerned with educational training, research and service provision.
- Results from major child health studies indicate that there is not, in any country, a systematic, continuous and comprehensive reporting of children's health, seen from the children's perspective and put into a social context.

- An overall objective of child public health would be to place the health of children in its full social, economic and political context.
- By work in interdisciplinary and multiprofessional teams, issues such as a healthy public policy for children, support for vulnerable groups, safe traffic planning, development of health indicators especially for children should be confronted.
- By finding allies and partners in professional and political spheres, it should be possible for child public health workers to act at the centre of children's health instead of at the periphery of medicine.

REFERENCES

1 Primary health care. Report of the international conference on primary health care. Geneva: World Health Organization, 1978
2 World Health Organization. Target for health for all. Copenhagen: WHO, 1985
3 World Health Organization. Targets for health for all. The health policy for Europe. Copenhagen: WHO, 1991
4 Public health in England. The report of the Committee of Inquiry into the Future Development of Public Health Function. London: HMSO, 1988
5 Köhler L. Public health renaissance and the role of school of public health. Eur J Public Health 1991; 1: 2–9
6 Ottawa Charter for Health Promotion. Health Promot 1986; 1(4): 3–5
7 Köhler L, Jakobsson G. Children's health and well-being in the Nordic countries. Clinics in Developmental Medicine No 98. Oxford: MacKeith Press, 1987
8 Köhler L, ed. Barn och barnfamiljer i Norden. En studie av välfärd, hälsa och livskvalitet (Children and children's families in the Nordic countries. A study of well-being, health and quality of life). Göteborg: Nordic School of Public Health, 1990: NHV-Rapport 1990: 1
9 Köhler L. Infant mortality: the Swedish experience. Annu Rev Public Health 1991; 12: 177–193
10 Köhler L, Jakobsson G. Children's health in Sweden. An overview for the 1991 Public Health Report. Stockholm: Swedish National Board of Health and Welfare, 1991

2. How can child health services contribute to a reduction in health inequalities in childhood?

T. Waterston

The persistence of inequalities in child health is among the greatest ills in our society and the reduction in the gap in death and morbidity rates between well-off and disadvantaged children should be among the top priorities of child health services. This chapter reviews the present state of knowledge on the extent of inequalities and the reasons, and examines how child health services can help raise all children's health to that of the healthiest.

THE EXTENT OF INEQUALITY IN HEALTH

Inequality in health may be defined as the difference in health status between the groups showing the highest and the lowest parameters in a society. There are problems with this definition — what groups are chosen, and what is health? The usual way of looking at differences ('variations' as they are described by the present Government) is by social class, which depends on the occupation of the head of household. Data are not generally available on income, which would be a better means of grouping; the variations within each social class are considerable. Another method, developed by Townsend et al,[1] uses variables derived from the Census which can be related to place of residence, e.g. unemployment, housing and the uptake of benefits.

The usual measures of health, namely mortality and morbidity rates, are actually disease measures because it is difficult to define health objectively. Ideally, measures of well-being, of nutritional status, of exercise levels, of smoking prevalence, of mental health and of family security should be used in preference to disease rates. Those that are available also show marked variation across society. Figures 2.1–2.5 show some of the major areas of inequality and the trends over the last 15 years. A useful statistic to remember is that if all children under 16 years of age had the same chances of survival as the children of doctors, lawyers and managers, then child mortality would fall by a quarter.[2]

Figure 2.1 shows mortality for 1–14-year-olds by social class in 1990, Fig. 2.2 shows low birthweight by social class, Fig. 2.3 shows pedestrian traffic accidents in the period 1979–1983, and Fig. 2.4 shows mortality from respiratory conditions in 1–14-year-olds over the same period. Similar findings are present for a host of other physical conditions as well as for

11

Per 100,000 population

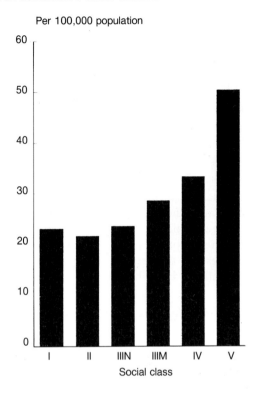

Fig. 2.1 Mortality (all causes) in children aged 1–14 years by social class, in England and Wales 1979–1980 and 1982–1983 (data represent 4-year averages). Source: OPCS DS 8. (Reproduced with permission from Woodroffe et al.[2])

behavioural problems and for risk factors such as dietary intake, smoking and unprotected sexual activity. Figure 2.5 shows the trends in poverty in children and the whole population between 1979 and 1987. Subsequent figures for the period 1990–1991 show poverty in 31% of children, and 24% of the whole population.

TRENDS IN INEQUALITIES IN HEALTH

Kumar[3] has shown that differentials in infant mortality widened in the 1980s for births within marriage. Evidence is less clear-cut for morbidity. Deteriorating dental caries has been described in the North of England, Wales and Scotland.[4,5] Trends towards increasing height among 5–11-year-old children had ceased by the period 1979–1986.[6] Obesity is increasing and social class differences are marked.[7] Dietary intakes of children from poor families have worsened since nutritionally balanced school meals have been replaced by free-choice cafeterias with an emphasis on 'fast foods'.[8]

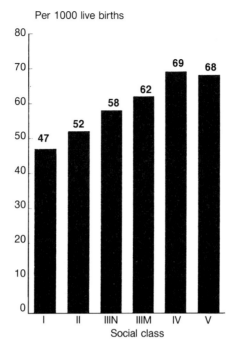

Fig. 2.2 Low birthweight by social class, in England and Wales 1990. Source: OPCS DH3/24. Births under 2500 g, within marriage only. (Reproduced with permission from Woodroffe et al.[2])

REASONS FOR INEQUALITIES IN CHILD HEALTH

The Black Report[9] considered four explanations for social inequalities in health, and these might all apply to children. They are: artefactual, social mobility, structural and lifestyle factors. The first asserts that the differences between occupational classes is a product of the way classes are defined, and may artificially exaggerate the differences. This reason may be discounted since other means of showing differences such as the Townsend Index demonstrates them to be as marked. Social mobility has been shown by Quick & Wilkinson[10] to make only a small contribution to the variation. Structural and lifestyle factors are now thought to be closely interrelated; i.e. a certain lifestyle is adopted by a family because of the environmental and economic constraints they live with. Exercise is not an easy option if the only sports facilities are in private clubs; 'healthy eating' is more expensive than cooking with filling but fatty foods; smoking is 'part of a complex array of coping strategies that women use when caring in low income and disadvantaged households'.[11] The major underlying reason for the persisting inequalities would seem to be child poverty. Figure 2.5 shows the trend in poverty for children and the whole population in the UK during 1979–1987. Latest figures show 31% of children living in families below half the average income.[12]

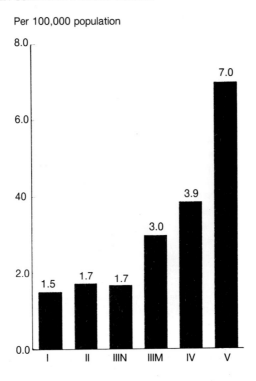

Fig. 2.3 Mortality from traffic collision with pedestrians aged 1–14 years, by social class, in England and Wales 1979–1980 and 1982–1983 (data represent 4-year averages). Source: OPCS DS 8. (Reproduced with permission from Woodroffe et al.[2])

Wise & Meyers[13] further analysed the reasons for disparities in child mortality and morbidity.

IS REDUCTION OF INEQUALITIES POSSIBLE?

The question must first be asked, is reduction in inequalities in health possible? Charlton[14] argues that inequalities in health are 'less a sign of deliberate failure to address deprivation, than an unintended consequence of success in expanding advantage'. He asserts that, because all societies demonstrate significant inequalities in health, inequality is not caused by deprivation or poverty but is a consequence of the distribution of social advantages. Charlton holds that health can be improved by making everyone richer, but redistribution of wealth is undesirable because this would make the well off less healthy. However, experience across Europe shows that life expectancy is strongly associated with income disparity and the highest rates occur in countries with the smallest gap between rich and poor. Power[15] suggests that the differences can be reduced by government policy. Quick & Wilkinson[10] take the opposite view to Charlton, arguing that the extent of

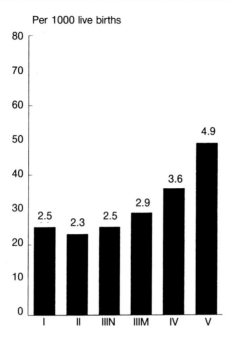

Per 1000 live births

Fig. 2.4 Mortality from respiratory conditions in children aged 1–14 years, by social class, in England and Wales 1979–1980 and 1982–1983. Source: OPCS DS 8. (Reproduced with permission from Woodroffe et al.[2])

inequality of income is a large part of the reason for the poor health shown by the deprived: 'Large differences in absolute income have little or no effect on mortality, but small differences in income distribution appear to have a large effect'. They draw attention to the 'psychological and social implications of income differences, of relative poverty and of having to live in conditions which are recognisably substandard'.

ROLE OF HEALTH SERVICES

There is much theory but little evidence available to show how child health services can reduce inequalities. Some might argue that it is not a clinician's role to reduce inequalities, that this is a political task. Wise & Meyers[13] confronted this view and their words are worth quoting.

Ultimately, it is the clinician who provides health services to poor children. However, the needs of these children can never fully be met by clinical management alone. In this setting, the role of the clinician is defined by the dual appreciation of medicine's efficacy and its inherent limitations. The emphasis of one to the exclusion of the other can be problematic. A total dependence on the provision of direct clinical service will not address the larger social forces that shape clinical need. Rejecting the importance of clinical contributions could

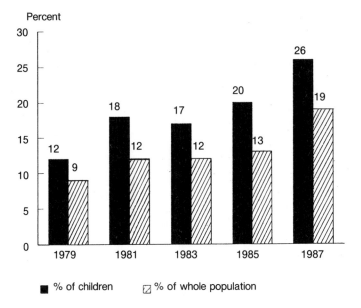

Fig. 2.5 Trend in children in poverty (living in households below half average income), Great Britain 1972–1987. Source: Oppenheim 1990. (Reproduced with permission from Woodroffe et al.[2])

preclude their many ameliorative effects and undermine efforts to bring about greater equity to their effective availability.

With Wise & Meyers, I believe that the paediatrician must work with others to challenge the determinants of poverty. The ways in which we can work towards greater health equity may be grouped as follows:

1. *Socioeconomic measures* aimed at poverty reduction.
   Means — data collection
   　　　　— collaboration with other organizations
   　　　　— advocacy
2. *Population-based health service measures* aimed at improving access to services. (This is a purchaser role.)
   Means — resource allocation
   　　　　— intersectoral collaboration
   　　　　— community development
   　　　　— 'Healthy cities' projects
   　　　　— data collection on deprivation indices
   　　　　— salaried GP services for deprived areas
3. *Client-based health service measures* aimed at increasing access. (This is a provider role.) .
   Means — siting and mode of provision of clinics
   　　　　— improved communication with consumers
   　　　　— targeting of preventive services

I have used the current 'purchaser/provider split' as a way of grouping the measures above. This is in recognition of the value of this scheme and of its likelihood to remain in operation for some years. I hope that it will always continue to be possible for paediatricians, who are working to benefit all children, to ignore these divisions and collaborate effectively with both purchasers (whether GPs or health authority) and providers of health services.

I will illustrate each of the above measures with practical examples.

Socioeconomic measures

There is evidence that government policies have increased economic differences and there is every reason to expect that government policies can reduce them. Paediatricians can exert pressure in this direction by ensuring good data collection, by collaboration with other organizations, and by advocacy. In other words, we research the nature and extent of inequalities, share our findings with others whose prime concern is the needs of children (e.g. the National Children's Bureau, the Health Visitors' Association, Child Poverty Action Group) and speak out in the public sphere without fear or favour.

Population-based health service measures

In the provider/purchaser split, the purchaser or commissioner of health services has the task of assessing health need in a given population. This task requires monitoring, policy-making and allocation of resources. In all these areas, the reduction of inequalities (or the assurance of equity) should be a major goal. Monitoring requires the collection of data which will show the extent of inequalities and trends. This should be on a small area basis. The inclusion of a deprivation indicator in routinely collected data would assist such monitoring. In this way, it is possible to review disparities in immunization uptake, in breast-feeding rates, in height at school entry, in weight in infancy, in infectious disease notification rates, and in accidents[16] as well as in mortality. Risk factor variables such as nutritional intakes in school children, smoking rates and alcohol intake, should also be routinely monitored. Table 2.1 lists the parameters which should be collected routinely and are related to deprivation. The use of deprivation indices has been fully discussed by Spencer & Janes.[17]

Information should also be collected from a community (see Harvey[18]). Harvey describes the Community Diagnosis Profile which includes service data, epidemiological data, socioeconomic and environmental data, behavioural and related data, competence and cultural data, and community perceptions. He calls the process 'democratized data gathering'.

Policy-making should flow from such a monitoring system. Policies would include resource allocation to areas of high need, interagency work and specific measures such as the development of safety equipment loan schemes;

Table 2.1 Data that should be collected routinely to monitor deprivation

Birth weight
Breast-feeding rates
Weight gain in infancy
Height at school entry
Smoking in 14-year-olds
Teenage conception rates
Accidental injury rates
Infectious disease notification rates
Mortality rates at different ages

these are dealt with below in the provider section. It is necessary that policies which make equity a key feature be inscribed in contracts between purchaser and providers. Resource allocation should be in relation to need and should unify health and social services. Judge & Mays[19] showed that health and social services departments are funded in quite different ways. The weighted capitation system used in the health service and introduced in 1990–1991 has many drawbacks, benefiting as it does London and areas with high proportions of the elderly; the standard spending assessment used by social services is allocated to local authorities in quite a different way. Judge & Mays recommend bringing together the different sources of funding into a unified weighted capitation system at a single level of aggregation.

Healthy cities

The healthy cities concept is based on the notion that health services alone cannot improve health but that in cooperation with other agencies (the so-called 'healthy alliances' with housing, education, transport, etc.) they can. Intersectoral collaboration is a key component of the World Health Organization's (WHO) 'Primary health care', as is community participation, both of which have been translated to an urban setting in the WHO healthy cities movement.[20] Implicit in 'healthy cities' is the aim to reduce health inequalities, particularly those related to environmental problems, e.g. child accidents (provision of safe play areas and traffic calming), malnutrition (provision of school meals), behaviour problems (provision of preschool child care). Lifestyle factors such as smoking and alcohol abuse can also be tackled by rigorous monitoring of under-age sales and the banning of smoking in public places, restaurants and schools.

The object of healthy cities is to make the city a healthier place to live in by collaboration between sectors and with local communities. If child injuries in the parts of the city with the highest rates could be brought down to the levels of those areas with the lowest rates, then inequality in this field would have been removed. Evaluation of healthy cities work at this level has not been carried out and needs to be. The key components of the healthy cities concept[20] are: assessment of health need; involvement of local people in planning; collaboration between local authority, health and voluntary sector in service development and health promotion; the development of healthy public policies.

Community development

Local efforts can confront serious health problems and indeed this is a principle of 'health cities'. Local health services can work with local people without the umbrella of 'health cities', and indeed must do so if health promotion is to have any effect. Community development is an effort to confront poverty and deprivation at local level by working with members of the local community, and relies on a policy of partnership and 'bottom-up' planning. As with the healthy cities movement, there has been little evaluation of the effect of community development on health inequalities. However, low self-esteem is an important part of the pathway between deprivation and ill-health, and self-esteem is enhanced in good community development projects.

Case studies

The following case studies illustrate how data collection, intersectoral collaboration and community development may be used to reduce or mitigate the effects of poverty on child health.

1. Breast-feeding

Breast-feeding is recognized to health promoting in infancy through the prevention of respiratory infections and gastroenteritis, the reduction of sudden infant death, and the reduction of maternal breast cancer (to name just a few). Yet there are wide variations in breast-feeding rates across the social classes together with a rapid fall-off in breast-feeding after birth which is also class-linked.[21] The reasons for the variations are multiple: lack of support from partners and relatives; lack of good examples in the local community; unawareness of health benefits of breast feeding; embarrassment over seeming to be different.

A breast-feeding promotion group was established which drew members from paediatrics, midwifery, health visiting, general practice, management and the voluntary sector.

Data collection. The group recognized that information was needed to examine the reasons for the rapid fall-off after birth and to monitor rates around the city. A medical student carried out a study on hospital practice which entailed questioning all midwives and health visitors in the city, as well as breast-feeding mothers. The study showed[22] that breast-fed babies were sometimes separated from their mother at night, offered water and complementary feeds after birth, and that midwives' views were not adequately in tune with a pro-breast-feeding policy.

The group obtained agreement from community information services to process manual data collected by health visitors on breast-feeding rates in their own case-load

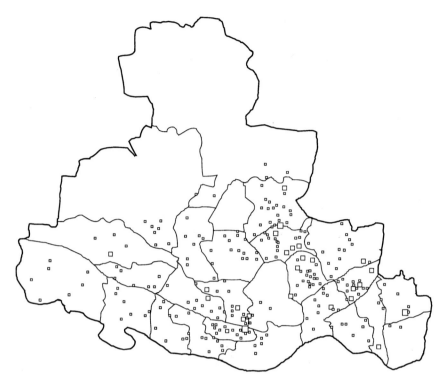

Fig. 2.6 Map showing distribution of breast-fed infants (birth cohort 1 April to 30 June 1993) at the time of health visitor's primary visit, by electoral ward within Newcastle upon Tyne. □, indicates one breast-fed infant. Where more than one breast-fed infant resides within a unit postcode, the size of the symbol is scaled up accordingly.

at birth, at 10 days and at 3 months. This data collection will not run continuously but for a 3-month period each year. The rates can be presented by GP practice or by locality (Fig. 2.6) and are fed back to the practice at the end of the survey period. The aim is to increase attention to low rates, to allow the evaluation of interventions, and to encourage the adoption of targets.

Intersectoral collaboration.   Breast-feeding cannot be enhanced by health services alone and the influences on practices are multiple. The group in Newcastle is developing two initiatives. The first is between disciplines in the health service to obtain a 'baby friendly' hospital award.[23] This entails collaboration between midwives, obstetrician, managers and voluntary groups to modify hospital practices towards those that are optimal to encourage breast-feeding. This is not an easy task as much lip service is paid to breast-feeding and customs are difficult to change. A start has been made by the introduction of a breast-feeding policy.

Two members of the breast-feeding promotion group addressed the women's issues subcommittee of the local council, which agreed to circulate the policy to all employees — with the aim of adopting it — and to all council premises. This would mean that breast-feeding mothers in libraries, recreation centres and swimming pools would find facilities available and encouragement to breast-feed their baby either in private or in public.

Community development. The group has addressed community support issues through the introduction of a La Leche League Peer Counsellor Scheme,[24] funded by the local children's charity. This scheme is aimed at localities with low breast-feeding rates and poor community support. Eight women with breast-feeding experience from a deprived area of Newcastle were given 3 months' training in breast-feeding technology and health education techniques. They will now act as counsellors for breast-feeding women in the locality, as health educators and as a vocal pressure group for breast-feeding. They are extremely enthusiastic and motivated. The effectiveness of their work in prolonging breast-feeding experience will be evaluated using the data collected by health visitors.

Expected outcome. More positive attitudes towards breast-feeding in the community; less rapid fall-off in breast feeding after birth; (later) increased breast-feeding rates.

2. Child injury prevention

Childhood accidents are the main cause of death in over-ones and also show marked social class variations, as was seen in Fig. 2.3. Variations are due mainly to environmental differences: lack of safety equipment in the home, lack of safe play areas in the street. Again, the health services alone can do little in injury prevention apart from education, which has been shown to be less effective than environmental modification in bringing about change.[25]

As part of the Healthy Cities Project in Newcastle, a child injury prevention group was set up, including a paediatrician, paediatric epidemiologist, health education officer, health visitor, relevant local authority departments and voluntary sector.

Data collection. It was apparent that good data collection was lacking so a monitoring system was established to identify accident risk by locality. In preschool children this involved surveys by health visitor on the availability of home safety equipment (stair gates, fireguards, cooker guards); in school children it included questionnaires on exposure to main roads on the way to school. Data were also collected from accident and emergency departments on injury events following accidents. Fig. 2.7 shows the map that was produced to illustrate the distribution of child accident risk around Newcastle.

At the same time a group of parents had been working with the health visitor on identifying local priorities and concerns. A major issue was heavy traffic on the main road which children crossed on the way to school. The parents carried out a survey here, the results of which are shown in Fig. 2.8.

Intersectoral collaboration. It has not proved easy to engage the local authority departments — particularly the roads department, which has its own priorities and sees itself as the expert in accident prevention. Collaboration began with educational exercises and workshops when members of the different departments worked together to reach shared objectives. A first real step towards collaboration will be the appointment of a person responsible both to the local authority and to the health authority for data collection on accidents and injuries (we distinguish these terms, since accidents may not always be preventable but injuries are). The feeling of the group is that pressure/advocacy to the roads department by local community members is likely to be more effective than pressure from the health authority. The present political climate is a constraint in that little funding is available for traffic restraint

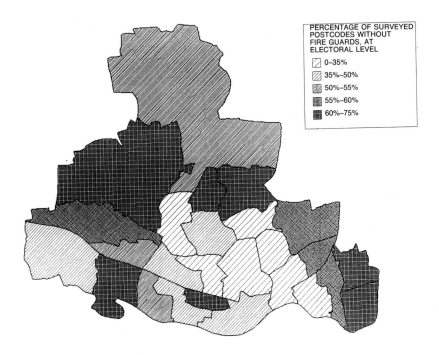

Fig. 2.7 Results of Woolfson studies (child accident risk data) for children aged 9 months, during 1990–1992 (Emamy N, Morphet C. Mapping child accident risk data. University of Northumbria, Newcastle, 1994. Data collected by Towner E, Jarvis S. Department of Child Health, University of Newcastle).

Q1 Safe crossing points on route to school

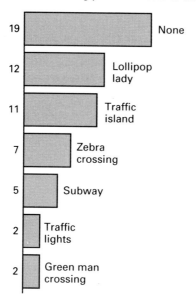

Q2 Main roads crossed on way to school

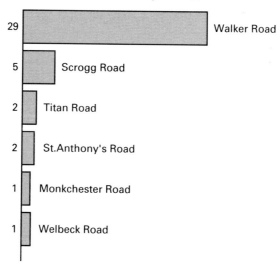

Fig. 2.8   Results of parental questionnaire.

schemes or cycle ways and there is no national support for targets to reduce car entry into cities or increase cycle usage.

Community development. The health visitor on the child injury prevention group attended several primary school parents' evenings to talk about childhood accidents. The parents expressed a wish to become active in prevention and set up a 'safety-setters' local injury prevention group. This group carried out the survey mentioned above, and also raised funds to start a safety equipment loan scheme. This scheme recognizes the difficulties many low income parents have in buying equipment. The group obtained a stock of fireguards, safety gates, cooker guards and other home safety equipment and loans it or sells it at cost price to local parents. There has been extensive demand for this equipment which is promoted and supplied from a local clinic.

Expected outcomes. The outcome of these schemes is fewer accidental injuries in children and a reduction in the social class divide. There should also be a greater awareness among parents about the causes of accidents, and greater confidence in their own ability to bring about change.

3. Provision of primary health care services

Many disadvantaged inner city areas have poor access to health care. The distribution of GP practices favours well-off areas and neglects deprived areas. As a result, inner city housing estates are likely to be served by many GPs and primary care teams. One estate in Newcastle which houses 1000 families is served by 25 GPs, but the nearest surgery (a single-handed one) is across a major dual carriage-way. Save the Children has been funding projects on the estate for some years, in collaboration with the health authority, Family Health Service Authority (FHSA), and social services. The Family Health and Community Project is designed to work with local people to improve the quality of primary health services. Two part-time health visitors are seconded to the project, and there is a steering group including locality health management, a paediatrician, social services management and the FHSA.

Community development. A drop-in centre has encouraged contact with local residents. A nearby children's centre, originally funded by Save the Children, allowed further opportunities for contacts with parents. Many activities developed on the Children's Centre premises.

Parents' concerns centred around crime, housing and accessibility of health services. Initiatives were developed in relation to the first two and there has been considerable investment in upgrading of housing and of the environment generally. The researcher with the project gathered a group of local parents to collect information specifically on health needs.

Data collection. The residents decided to carry out a questionnaire study on health which would be completed by every household on the estate (a sample question is given in Table 2.2). The survey was extensively advertised using posters. The title used — 'Do you want a doctor on the estate?' — might seem biased to an epidemiologist but was insisted on by the residents. It reflects their wish for curative as well as preventive services on the estate (not unreasonably). Some of the key results from the questionnaire are given in Table 2.3.

Table 2.2 A sample question from a housing estate residents' questionnaire study on health

25. Would you do any of these things if you or your children were ill and you couldn't get to the surgery? (for example, upset stomach, colds, headaches):

Try and treat the problem myself

Call the doctor out

Get something from the chemist

Go to the accident and emergency department at the hospital

Ask the health visitor's advice

Ask the nurse's advice

Ask someone else's advice

(please say who) ....

....

Table 2.3 Respondents were asked if they wanted any of the following services on the estate

Service	Number	% who said yes
Somewhere to get treatment for small cuts, bumps, sprains etc.	296	53
Health information	241	43
Baby Clinic	296	53
Ante Natal Care	139	25
Contraception Service	185	33
Health Services for Women (e.g. smears)	227	40
Chiropody	218	39
Alternative medicines/therapies	159	28
Dentist	257	46
Optician	268	48
Nurse who could prescribe	306	54
Counselling (e.g. advice, debt, bereavement)	197	35
Prescription collection service	298	53

Intersectoral collaboration. There are quite close working relationships between local councillors, housing department, social services and FHSA plus health authority, together with local people on the estate, although these are more at the level of coordination than collaboration. It is hoped that an innovative interdisciplinary health approach will be adopted on the lines of the Peckham Clinic in London, with all needs being addressed by staff working from common premises at the end of 1994, the local NHS trust is advertising for a salaried GP to work on the estate. This is a novel concept but in tune with locally expressed needs.

Expected outcomes. A locally based primary care team; greater user satisfaction with health services; (perhaps) fewer out of hours calls to GPs.

Making services more accessible

As Whitehead pointed out,[26] the principle of access for everyone as of right was a lynchpin of the National Health Service from the beginning. In this section I shall look at the role of the clinician in making his or her services more accessible. Whether or not this will make a difference to inequalities is not known. However, accessibility is an essential principle in ensuring an equitable service and there are barriers to access at present. The ingredients of improved access are quality issues which should be monitored in contracts; there should also be a means of obtaining user feedback to establish the degree of satisfaction. The main issues I wish to discuss are language and communication, the siting/timing of clinics, and targeting of services to those in need.

Language and communication

Communication difficulties abound in health care and are a consequence of medical mystique, medical language and class barriers. By medical mystique I mean the distrust (built into doctors' training) in communicating effectively on medical issues. Sanders[27] explains the reasons why doctors have not wished to divulge the secrets of their profession. Maintaining secrecy gave them the monopoly of marketing their commodity of health care. Many doctors still are not happy with a policy of complete openness of medical communication.

Even after dispensing with the mystique, we are stuck with a language that is impenetrable to the non-cognoscenti (this is part of the mystique too). This language is particularly difficult for people with poor literacy skills. Many words, even simple ones like 'lateral' and 'medial', are not in ordinary usage. We find it hard to translate and often do not feel it necessary to do so.

Class barriers remain considerable between doctors and their patients. Most doctors are middle class, and do not share the same values and culture as 'working class' patients. From the other side, lower socioeconomic group patients are anxious about doctors' authoritarian approach and sometimes judgemental attitude. They are uncomfortable in their presence and find their language almost impossible to understand.

How can the situation be improved, to make health care more accessible to patients of all backgrounds? Doctors should share information openly; they should use simple language, and test out patients' understanding of their explanation; they should learn about cultural and class values, and appreciate the difficulties families face in penetrating the health service. These points are equally if not more important to consider for families from ethnic minorities, who often suffer the abuse of racism as well as poverty.

There are tools which can improve communication. The personal health record[28] is one: it places an onus on doctors and other health workers to share information more openly, and in comprehensible language. Another is to send copies of hospital discharge or outpatient letters to parents.[29] Parents' understanding is increased, and the medical mystique reduced, by this simple method.

Siting and timing of clinics

Outpatient clinics can be difficult to access because of siting and timing. A hospital clinic may require a journey of 2 hours and a whole morning or afternoon, and for parents with low income and limited child care facilities this is not possible. An afternoon clinic may clash with school collection time for older children and a single parent may not easily make alternative arrangements.

Doctors who wish to improve access to their clinics should consider alternative venues: the GP surgery, or a clinic near the home. There is a lower proportion of non-attenders at such clinics than at hospital, and the opportunity to discuss management with the GP is an asset. Clinics should be timed to fit in with school times and an occasional out of hours session to accommodate working parents is much appreciated.

CONCLUSIONS

Inequalities in child health are severe and increasing and are a blot on our society. Means are available to reduce them through political means and through health service measures. Key principles are healthy public policy, intersectoral collaboration, and working with communities. Health professionals also need to listen carefully to parents and to communicate effectively in simple straightforward language.

REFERENCES

1 Townsend P, Phillimore P, Beattie A. Health and deprivation: inequality and the north. London: Croom Helm, 1987
2 Woodroffe C, Glickman M, Barker M, Power C. Children, teenagers and health — the key data. Buckingham: Open University Press, 1993
3 Kumar V. Poverty and inequality in the UK. The effects on children. London: National Children's Bureau, 1993
4 Carmichael CL, Rugg-Gunn A, Ferrell RS. The relationship between fluoridation, social class and caries experience in 5 yr old children in Newcastle and Northumberland in 1987. Br Dental J 1989; 167: 57–61.
5 Department of Health. On the state of the public health 1990. London: HMSO 1991
6 Chinn S, Rona RJ, Price CE. The secular trend in the height of primary school children in England and Scotland 1972–79 and 1979–86. Ann Hum Biol 1989; 16: 387–395
7 National Children's Bureau. Investing in the future: child health 10 yrs after the Court Report. London: National Children's Bureau, 1987
8 White J, Cole-Hamilton I, Dibb S. The nutritional case for school meals. London: School Meals Campaign, 1992
9 Department of Health and Social Security. Inequalities in health: report of a research working group (the Black Report). London: DHSS, 1980
10 Quick A, Wilkinson R. Income and health. London: Socialist Health Association, 1991
11 Blackburn C, Graham H. Smoking among working class mothers. Coventry: University of Warwick, 1991
12 National Children's Homes. The NCH Factfile 1993. London: National Children's Homes, 1993
13 Wise PH, Meyers A. Poverty and child health. Pediatr Clin North Am 1988; 35: 1169–1185
14 Charlton B. Is inequality bad for the national health? Lancet 1994; 343: 221–222
15 Power C. Medicine in Europe: health and social inequality in Europe. Br Med J 1994; 308: 1153–1156
16 Sharples PM, Storey A, Aynsley-Green A, Eyre JA. Causes of fatal childhood accidents involving head injury in Northern Region 1979–86. Br Med J 1990; 301: 1193–1197
17 Spencer N, Janes H, eds. Uses and abuses of deprivation indices. Proceedings of a conference. Coventry: University of Warwick, 1994
18 Harvey J. Assessing health needs for children. In: Waterston T, ed. Perspectives in social disadvantage and child health. Andover: Intercept, 1993
19 Judge K, Mays N. Equity in the NHS: allocating resources for health and social care in England. Br Med J 1994; 308: 1363–1366
20 Ashton J. Healthy cities. Milton Keynes: Open University Press, 1992
21 White A, Freeth S, O'Brien M. Infant feeding 1990. London: HMSO, 1990
22 Beeken S, Waterston T. Health service support of breast feeding — are we practising what we preach? Br Med J 1992; 305: 285–287
23 Waterston T, Davies J. Could hospitals do more to encourage breast feeding? Br Med J 1993; 307; 1437–1438
24 Peer counsellor programme. La Leche League of Great Britain, 1992
25 Powles JW, Gifford S. Health of nations: lessons from Victoria, Australia. Br Med J 1993; 306: 125–127

26 Whitehead M. Who cares about equity in the NHS? Br Med J 1994; 308: 1284–1287
27 Sanders D. The struggle for health. London: Macmillan, 1985
28 Macfarlane A. Personal health records held by parents. Arch Dis Child 1992; 67: 571–572
29 Rylance G. Patients' right to know. Br Med J 1990; 300: 608–609

3. New developments in SIDS: the case of the back-to-sleep campaign

R. Gilbert

Over the past 5 years, there has been a remarkable fall in the number of babies dying of sudden infant death syndrome (SIDS) in many Western industrialized countries. In England and Wales, for instance, the annual number of SIDS victims dropped by nearly 70%, falling from 1597 in 1988 to 531 in 1992[1,2] (Table 3.1), a dramatic reversal of previous trends. Altogether incidence of SIDS in England and Wales fell from 2.30/1000 live births to 0.77/1000 live births per year in this period. Equally marked reductions have been observed in Scotland,[3] New Zealand,[4] Australia,[5] The Netherlands,[6] Norway,[7] Denmark[8] and Ireland.[9] SIDS is still the biggest killer of young babies in these countries, and such an extraordinary improvement prompts the question 'why?'.

All the evidence points to the dramatic success of the 'back-to-sleep' campaign, the advice now given to parents to avoid the prone sleeping position for their infants.[10] That such a major and simple change in infant care practice could have such a marked effect on infant mortality is unprecedented in modern industrialized countries.

Table 3.1 SIDS victims by age in England and Wales, 1987–1992

Year	Numbers of SIDS victims (incidence*)		Percentage of all SIDS under 1 year			SIDS as proportion of all post-neonatal deaths (%)	Male/female ratio
			< 1 month	1–5 months	6–11 months		
1987	1528	(2.24)	5.0	81.3	13.7	53	1.43
1988	1597	(2.30)	5.2	80.2	14.6	53	1.57
1989	1337	(1.93)	5.4	81.6	13.0	50	1.50
1990	1202	(1.70)	6.5	80.2	13.3	48	1.44
1991	1008	(1.44)	6.2	79.0	14.9	45	1.60
1992	531	(0.77)	11.3	72.7	16.0	30	1.68
Decline (%) 1988–1992	67		23	70	63		

Data from refs 1, 2.
*SIDS deaths under 1 year of age per 1000 live births recorded as principal cause of death or mentioned anywhere on death certificate.

In this chapter, the progress of the campaign will be examined in detail, the evidence which led to the launch of campaigns in the UK and in other countries will be reviewed and the evidence for a causal link between such advice and the reduction in SIDS incidence will be discussed.

PRONE SLEEPING POSITION AND THE RISK OF SIDS

The evidence that sleeping prone is a major risk factor for SIDS came entirely from observational epidemiological studies. Nineteen case-control studies and one cohort study in eight different countries showed a three- to nine-fold increased risk of SIDS in babies who slept prone compared with those who slept on their side or supine.[11-26] Not all these studies have passed without criticism. Among the shortcomings were: inappropriate choice of control babies; recording of usual sleeping position rather than position put down or found; and recall bias.[14,27-29] Nevertheless, an association between prone sleeping and SIDS has been observed so frequently and consistently in so many different settings that a causal relationship is highly likely — especially since this association persists after allowing for confounding factors[22-24] and there is a dose effect with intermediate risk associated with side sleeping.[29,30]

There has been no controlled intervention trial to establish the risk of SIDS associated with different sleeping positions and the link is based entirely upon observational studies. Yet the observational evidence is so powerful that such a trial is no longer ethical, and so well-publicized[4,29] that it is no longer feasible.

Just how prone sleeping might lead to death remains unknown, but there are two principal areas of hypothesis. The first is the suggestion that diminished heat loss in the prone position, particularly in babies whose heads are covered,[30] has an effect on central respiratory control and increases the likelihood of prolonged apnoea. The second is that death may be caused by obstruction of the respiratory tract, either of the upper respiratory tract or of the large airways. In babies nursed prone it has been suggested that the upper respiratory tract may be obstructed when posterior movement of the mandible diminishes the posterior pharyngeal space.[31] Alternatively, particularly in infants with minor respiratory tract infections, it may be that partial upper respiratory tract obstruction is exacerbated by partial nasal obstruction in the prone position, creating negative pressure proximally and collapse of the large airways.[32] Recently, evidence has been put forward that dummies might provide protection against SIDS, although this has yet to be confirmed by other studies. It may be that dummies keep the tongue forward — thus helping to maintain airway patency by improving upper airway muscle tone — or they may reduce gastro-oesophageal reflux which is associated with apnoea (although gastro-oesophageal reflux has not been shown to be associated with SIDS).[33]

Other hypotheses about the mechanism for SIDS are reported frequently,[34-36] but few directly address the importance of the prone position.

RISKS AND BENEFITS FOR THE INFANT POPULATION

Any advice to the public about sleeping position must be based entirely on a careful assessment of the risks and benefits for the infant population. The potential benefits can be estimated by calculating the percentage reduction in SIDS incidence that might be achieved by avoiding prone sleeping, known as the 'population attributable risk'. Prior to the publicity about the risk of sleeping prone, the prevalence in different areas of prone sleeping among young infants ranged from 25% to 68%.[14] Assuming that the association between prone sleeping and SIDS is causal, the estimated population attributable risk for different countries, calculated from a variety of studies, has ranged from 38% to 82%.[22-24,26]

The perceived risks associated with the supine sleeping position for babies born at term are: death due to aspiration of gastric contents, gastro-oesophageal reflux[37] and upper respiratory tract obstruction in infants with mandibular hypoplasia.[29] Worldwide, infants most commonly sleep supine[38] whereas the prone position had been adopted by Western industrialized countries over the last 20-30 years (Table 3.2). In societies where babies are nursed supine, there is no known evidence of a higher infant mortality due to aspiration, and many such deaths occur in babies who slept prone.[38]

On a population basis, the balance of risks and benefits is clearly in favour of the supine sleeping position for the majority of infants after the first month of life. However, in some babies the benefits of sleeping prone may outweigh the risk of SIDS. These include: preterm babies and low birthweight newborns;[37,42] newborns with severe respiratory difficulty; term babies with severe gastro-oesophageal reflux; and babies with mandibular hypoplasia.[29]

HEALTH ADVICE ABOUT INFANT SLEEPING POSITION

One reason for the marked prevalence of the prone sleeping position for babies in Western industrial societies was the advice given to parents by health professionals in the late 1960s and early 1970s to nurse babies this way. This advice probably originated in the discovery that preterm infants benefited from this sleeping position.[24,43] What was shown to be good for preterm babies was assumed to be good for full-term babies too, but there was no evidence whatsoever to show that this is so — and the benefit of hindsight shows otherwise.

This time, health professionals have been much more careful before advising parents to nurse their babies supine. The 'back-to-sleep' campaigns in many countries (New Zealand,[44] the UK,[29] Norway,[7] Denmark[8] and The Netherlands[6]) have been based on consistent findings from a number of studies in different settings published in peer-reviewed journals. Moreover, advice about avoidance of the prone sleeping position has been issued only after a systematic assessment of the potential risks and benefits.[29]

The supine sleeping position was first advocated publicly in 1987 in a lecture by De Jonge when he reported the results of The Netherlands

Table 3.2   SIDS incidence and prevalence of prone sleeping among young infants in different countries

Country (and reference)	SIDS incidence (per 1000 live births)	Prevalence of prone sleeping in infants (%)
Avon (UK)		
1987–1989[26]	3.5	59
1990–1991	1.7	27
1992[29]	0.3[45]	2
The Netherlands		
1969[24,39]	0.4	10
1977	1.2	
1985[6]	1.1	62 (1982–1987)
1986	1.0	63 (1985–1987)
1987	0.9	56
1988	0.6	27
1989	0.7	
1990	0.6	16
1991	0.4	9
New Zealand[40]		
1985	4.2	
1986	4.0	42
1987	4.3	
1988	3.7	
1989	3.9	
1990	3.1	2 (1989–1990)
1991	2.1	
Norway[7]		
1970	1.1	10
1985	2.6	55
1989	2.5	54
1991–1992	1.3	31

*Retrospective data based on 24 371 families.

case-control study.[6] At that time there was supportive evidence from four other case-control studies,[11,12,17,18] giving similar findings regarding the risk of SIDS associated with the prone position. In the UK, the findings of the Avon case-control study[25] were published in June 1990 amid a great deal of national media interest. Parents in Avon were also advised by health professionals at this time to avoid the prone sleeping position and avoid heavy wrapping for their infants. However, it was not until 16 months later, after the publication of similar findings from New Zealand in February 1991[23] and a highly influential TV documentary on the subject in October 1991, that the UK government launched their national back-to-sleep campaign in November 1991.[29]

In New Zealand, a back-to-sleep campaign was launched in February 1991 but was preceded by national publicity in 1989 and 1990.[4] Other European countries have since publicly advised parents to put their infants supine, and in the USA the American Academy of Pediatrics voted to recommend avoiding the prone position in April 1993.[45]

However, despite the caution with which national back-to-sleep campaigns were launched, very little has been done to systematically monitor their progress. Information on the prevalence of the prone position in the infant population before and after the publicity campaign is only available for Avon in the UK, for The Netherlands and for New Zealand, and also in retrospectively collected data for Norway (Table 3.2). All of these places show there has been a marked drop in the proportion of infants sleeping prone. There has also been a marked fall in the incidence of SIDS. The relationship between these changes is discussed below.

OTHER RISK FACTORS FOR SIDS

When assessing how far the change in prone position might account for the fall in SIDS incidence, it is necessary to examine changes in other risk factors for SIDS. Consistent associations, for instance, have been established between SIDS and male sex, intrauterine growth retardation, preterm birth, poor socioeconomic status, young maternal age, multiple birth and short interpregnancy interval.[46] The prevalence of these factors changes little from year to year. But associations have also been established with a range of much more variable environmental factors besides prone sleeping position. Particularly important among these is maternal smoking which has been consistently associated with SIDS, but there may also be links with heavy wrapping, infection, bottle feeding or bed sharing. The contribution of any one risk factor to the fall in SIDS incidence depends on the associated relative risk for SIDS, the prevalence of the factor in the young infant population and the change in prevalence.

Maternal smoking

Maternal smoking has consistently been found to at least double the risk of SIDS in 14 studies[23,28,47-57] conducted in eight different countries. Of these, two prospective cohort studies[49,50] and four case-control studies[23,47,48,53] took some account of confounding due to social factors, preterm birth and low birthweight. The risk of SIDS increased with the number of cigarettes smoked by the mother[23,49,50,53,56] and if both parents smoked.[47,53] The effect of maternal smoking appears to be highest in infants under 10 weeks of age.[50,53] The population attributable risk for maternal smoking has been estimated to be as high as 40%.[23]

Infection

Despite earlier suspicions, no clear association has yet been established between SIDS and presence of bacterial or viral pathogens.[47,58] Interpretation of findings from many case-control studies has been made harder by possible selection bias of cases and controls, incomparability of microbiological samples and lack of attention to potential confounding factors.[59-62] In a UK study,[59] differences in sampling techniques probably led to an overestimation of the difference in virus prevalence which was 16% and 8%, respectively, in SIDS and live control babies ($P > 0.05$). However, even if this difference did represent a causal association, eradication of virus infections in infancy would lead only to an estimated 7% reduction in SIDS mortality.[47]

Bottle feeding

Overall, there is suggestive but inconsistent evidence for an increased risk of SIDS in bottle-fed babies. Of 11 studies[23,52,55,63-69] which found a two- to three-fold increased risk of SIDS in bottle-fed babies, only three[52,63,70] took account of confounding due to social factors, preterm birth, low birthweight and maternal smoking. The New Zealand study demonstrated that this association persisted throughout the first 4 months of life. The risk of SIDS was increased in babies bottle fed from birth and in those who were changed from breast to bottle later on.[70] Seven case-control studies[22,24,71-75] found no association. In New Zealand, the population attributable risk for not breast feeding at hospital discharge has been estimated to be 22%.[70]

Heavy wrapping

Only three case-control studies have investigated the association between the thermal insulation of clothing and bedding and SIDS.[25,76,77] Overall, the evidence for an effect is inconclusive. One study found an increased risk of SIDS in babies over 10 weeks of age who were heavily wrapped.[25] The effect of heavy wrapping was further increased in babies who were found prone or had viruses identified in the upper respiratory tract or gastrointestinal tract.[59] A subsequent study in the same geographical area conducted after publicity about the risks associated with the prone position and heavy wrapping found no association.[77] In an Australian study,[76] the risk of SIDS increased with the degree of wrapping for a given room temperature.

One possible explanation for these inconsistent findings is that heavy wrapping is associated with an increased risk of SIDS only when other thermal stressors such as the prone position are present. Heat loss is reduced in the prone compared with the supine position[30] and physiological studies have shown that nocturnal body temperature is higher in babies over 12 weeks old who are heavily wrapped and sleep prone.[78] However, detection of this 'interaction' between heavy wrapping and the prone position by epidemiological studies requires much larger sample sizes than have hitherto been studied.

Bed sharing

Evidence for an association between bed sharing and SIDS is weak. Laboratory studies[79] have indicated possible advantages of mother–infant bed sharing for the development of respiratory and temperature rhythms but these have been based on infants least at risk of SIDS studied in an artificial environment. The relevance of these findings for SIDS is unclear. In contrast, a recent epidemiological study showed an increased risk of SIDS in babies who shared their bed with another person, particularly if the mother smoked.[80]

These results require cautious interpretation. As bed sharing is highly culturally determined,[81] an apparent association may be due to residual confounding by other social and cultural factors.[82] Furthermore, interactions such as that detected between maternal smoking and bed sharing[80] will arise by chance if enough interactions are examined.

EARLY RISE IN SIDS

SIDS incidence rose steadily in England and Wales throughout the 1970s after SIDS became a registerable cause of death in 1971 (Fig. 3.1, Table 3.3). However, this rise in incidence may have been largely attributable to

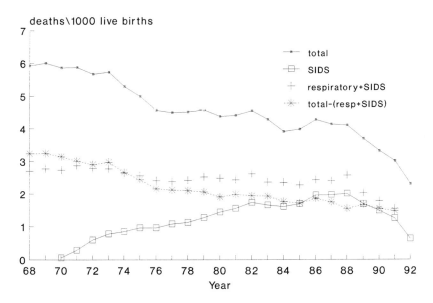

Fig. 3.1 Postneonatal deaths by cause: England and Wales, 1968–1992. Data from refs 1, 29. SIDS recorded as main underlying cause. Key: ▣, total postneonatal deaths; ▢, postneonatal SIDS; +, postneonatal non-SIDS respiratory deaths and SIDS combined; *, all postneonatal deaths excluding SIDS and non-SIDS respiratory deaths. (Reproduced with permission from Gilbert.[10])

Table 3.3 Actual data given in Fig. 3.1: postneonatal deaths by cause, England and Wales

Patient	Year	Deaths/1000 live births			
		Total	SIDS	Non-SIDS resp + SIDS	Total − (SIDS + resp)
1	1968	5.93		2.7	3.23
2		6.01		2.77	3.24
3	1970	5.87	0.06	2.73	3.14
4		5.88	0.29	2.87	3.01
5	1972	5.68	0.6	2.78	2.9
6		5.74	0.78	2.77	2.97
7	1974	5.3	0.85	2.64	2.66
8		5	0.96	2.56	2.44
9	1976	4.57	0.96	2.41	2.16
10		4.5	1.08	2.38	2.12
11	1978	4.52	1.13	2.42	2.1
12		4.58	1.27	2.52	2.06
13	1980	4.38	1.44	2.48	1.9
14		4.41	1.55	2.43	1.98
15	1982	4.55	1.73	2.61	1.94
16		4.29	1.65	2.36	1.93
17	1984	3.91	1.6	2.35	1.76
18		3.98	1.69	2.27	1.71
19	1986	4.28	1.96	2.43	1.85
20		4.14	1.97	2.4	1.74
21	1988	4.11	2.01	2.57	1.54
22		3.69	1.69	2.03	1.66
23	1990	3.32	1.48	1.78	1.54
24		3.01	1.25	1.54	1.47
25	1992	2.3	0.63		

diagnostic transfer from respiratory causes to SIDS as these rates combined remained relatively constant. This change in certification practice makes it difficult to examine the effect of an increase in prone sleeping during the same period.

However, evidence from some countries suggests that a rise in SIDS incidence similar to that observed in the UK may have been partly due to an increase in infant prone sleeping. Prone sleeping was promoted from the early 1970s in Europe and New Zealand,[39,43] although in the USA prone had been the predominant infant sleeping position for most of the century.[83] From 1970 onwards, the rise in SIDS incidence was associated with an increase in total 1–5-month mortality in New Zealand and Sweden which may have been due to an increase in unexplained deaths.[84] Furthermore, data from The Netherlands[5] and Norway[6] have shown a close correlation between the rise in prevalence of prone sleeping and increase in SIDS incidence from the early 1970s.

FALL IN SIDS INCIDENCE

In England and Wales, SIDS incidence stabilized in the mid-1980s and has fallen steadily since 1988, predominantly in the postneonatal age group (Table 3.1). Postneonatal incidence plotted on a logarithmic scale (Fig. 3.2, Table 3.4) shows a steady proportional decline of 14.5% per year between 1988 and 1991. This decline is unlikely to be explained by diagnostic transfer because postneonatal mortality from causes other than SIDS has also declined, albeit more slowly.

Had the fall of 14.5% per year continued, the predicted incidence in 1992 would have been 1.16/1000 live births. The actual incidence was 0.68/1000 live births, 41% below that predicted. This sharp fall in postneonatal SIDS incidence in 1992 was not evident in other causes of postneonatal mortality and is therefore likely to have been due to changes in risk factors specific for SIDS. In Scotland, postneonatal SIDS incidence declined slightly in 1990 but dropped substantially in 1991 and in 1992 in contrast to the gradual decline in other causes of postneonatal mortality over the same period (Fig. 3.2, Table 3.4).

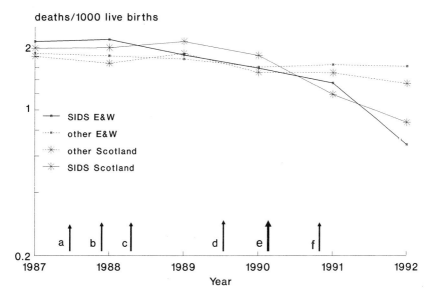

Fig. 3.2 Postneonatal mortality trends and publicity about sleeping position. Data from refs 1, 3, 29, 85. SIDS recorded as main underlying cause or mentioned anywhere on death certificate. Key: a, Hong Kong experience reported June 1988;[86] b, anecdotal findings in Australia reported November 1988;[12] c, Dutch case-control study published March 1989;[21] d, Avon case-control study published July 1990;[25] e, publication of New Zealand study findings, February 1991;[23] f, National back-to-sleep campaign launched by Chief Medical Officer, November 1991.[29] E, England; W, Wales. (Modified from Gilbert.[10])

Table 3.4   Actual data given in Fig 3.2: postneonatal mortality trends

Patient	Year	Deaths/1000 live births			
		SIDS in England and Wales	Other causes, England and Wales	SIDS in Scotland	Other causes, Scotland
1	1987	2.13	1.87	1.98	1.81
2	1988	2.18	1.82	1.99	1.68
3	1989	1.84	1.76	2.13	1.87
4	1990	1.59	1.61	1.83	1.52
5	1991	1.35	1.65	1.19	1.51
6	1992	0.68	1.62	0.87	1.34

CORRELATION WITH PUBLICITY ABOUT RISK FACTORS

From 1988 onwards, information about the risks associated with the prone position was published in the medical journals (Fig. 3.2, Table 3.4) but it is not known if health professionals in the UK changed their advice to parents as a result. There is little doubt that the official government back-to-sleep campaign which began in 1991 had a strong effect on public knowledge of the risks associated with prone sleeping[29] and coincided with a sharp decline in the number of SIDS cases.

The problem is to assess just how much this publicity influenced the decline in SIDS incidence. First, underlying trends in incidence are partly obscured by random year-to-year variation. This is particularly true of the rates for Scotland, which are based on fewer deaths. This may be why SIDS incidence departs from pre-existing trends 1 year earlier in Scotland than in England and Wales. Secondly, it may not be possible to date precisely the onset of effective publicity. A recent retrospective study showed that health visitors in Scotland started to advise avoiding the prone position long before the official government back-to-sleep campaign.[87]

A further problem is to identify just what advice has been effective. The main advice in all recent risk reduction campaigns has been to avoid the prone sleeping position, but sometimes parents have also been advised to avoid smoking and heavy wrapping, and to breast feed.[8,29,44]

Nevertheless, a substantial fall in SIDS incidence has occurred in several countries following all publicity campaigns which included advice about sleeping position.[6-9,12,26] It seems unlikely that these declines are simply due to increased parental vigilance; a previous intervention study to improve infant care by parents failed to alter pre-existing trends in SIDS incidence.[88] So there is at least a strong possibility that advice to avoid prone sleeping has been effective.

CORRELATION WITH CHANGE IN PREVALENCE OF RISK FACTORS IN POPULATION

The best evidence for a link between risk factor publicity and the decline in SIDS incidence comes from studies in New Zealand, The Netherlands and Avon, UK. Here, data on the prevalence of environmental risk factors were collected before and after the decline in SIDS incidence[6,27,88] (Table 3.2). The data showed that only the reduction in the prevalence of prone sleeping was of sufficient magnitude to account for the fall in SIDS incidence.[40,77] In The Netherlands, a slight fall in maternal smoking may have had a marginal effect on SIDS incidence,[39] but in England the prevalence of smoking has remained static among women of childbearing age.[89]

Yet despite this strong correlation between the fall in SIDS incidence and the prevalence of prone sleeping, such studies provide intrinsically weak evidence on which to base public health action. It is never possible to rule out some other 'cause' for the decline in incidence, and the original case-control studies linking sleeping position and SIDS remain the best justification for advice on sleeping position.

CHANGING CHARACTERISTICS OF THE SIDS POPULATION

In the UK, the decrease in SIDS incidence has been most marked in the postneonatal age range (Table 3.1). Among neonates, the fall in incidence has been 23%, compared with 70% in the 1–5-month age group and 63% in 6–11-month old infants (Table 3.1). The proportional decrease in the number of deaths, shown on a log scale comparing the mean annual number of deaths for 1986–1990 with the number in 1992 for England and Wales (unpublished data provided by the Office of Population Censuses and Surveys (OPCS)) (Fig. 3.3, Table 3.5), appears to be remarkably consistent throughout the postneonatal age range. The decline is similar for both boys and girls and persists even after 6 months of age when most infants would be able to change their position themselves. This may be because infants get into the habit of sleeping in one position even when they can change if they want to.

There also appears to have been a small but not significant increase in the ratio of boys to girls in SIDS victims in 1992, but it is too early to see whether this is a continuing trend (Table 3.1). Surprisingly, perhaps, the fall in SIDS incidence in the UK among babies born to mothers of Asian origin is similar to that among babies born to UK-born mothers (Fig. 3.4, Table 3.6, unpublished data from OPCS). Such groups are widely thought to traditionally nurse infants supine.[90,91] This emphasizes the need for more information on the change in risk factors in different groups.

From the point of view of paediatric clinical practice, sudden unexpected infant deaths are now more likely to be explained and efforts to look for causes such as metabolic, infection and non-accidental injury should be increased.

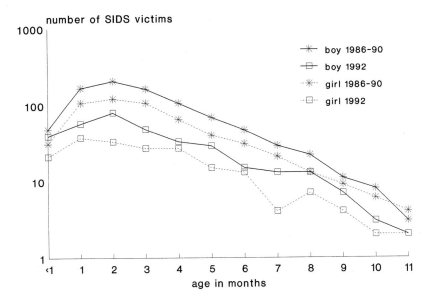

Fig. 3.3 Decline in the number of SIDS victims in England and Wales according to age and sex. Unpublished data from OPCS, showing mean annual number of SIDS deaths in 1986–1990 compared with the number of SIDS deaths in 1992 (plotted on a logarithmic scale to show proportional decline).

Table 3.5 Actual data given in Fig. 3.3: decline in SIDS in England and Wales according to age and sex

Patient	Age (months)	No. of SIDS victims			
		Boy 1986–1990	Boy 1992	Girl 1986–1990	Girl 1992
1	<1	48	39	31	21
2	1	167	57	107	37
3	2	206	80	121	33
4	3	163	48	107	27
5	4	106	33	65	27
6	5	69	29	40	15
7	6	47	15	31	13
8	7	29	13	21	4
9	8	22	13	13	7
10	9	11	7	9	4
11	10	8	3	6	2
12	11	3	2	4	2

PUBLIC HEALTH ACTION

Irrefutable evidence that prone sleeping causes SIDS is not available. The mechanism is not understood and no intervention study has yet been

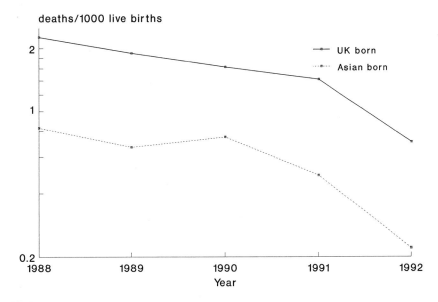

Fig 3.4 Postneonatal SIDS mortality in babies born to UK-born and Asian-born mothers. Unpublished data from OPCS. Asian-born includes mothers born in Bangladesh, India, Pakistan and East Africa.

Table 3.6 Actual data given in Fig. 3.4: postneonatal SIDS mortality in babies born to UK- and Asian-born mothers

Patient	Year	Deaths/1000 live births	
		UK-born mothers (number)	Asian-born mothers (number)
1	1988	2.26 (1382)	0.83 (28)
2	1989	1.9 (1154)	0.67 (22)
3	1990	1.63 (1020)	0.75 (25)
4	1991	1.42 (878)	0.49 (16)
5	1992	0.71 (429)	0.22 (7)

conducted. Public health recommendations to avoid prone sleeping in young infants have been based largely on evidence from case-control and cohort studies; on balance, the potential benefits of supine sleeping for SIDS prevention have been considered to outweigh possible adverse effects, except for babies with severe mandibular hypoplasia or severe symptomatic gastro-oesophageal reflux.

In many countries, recommendations in favour of supine sleeping have been widely publicized. In the UK, there is undoubtedly scope for further public health action to reduce environmental risk factors for SIDS. Many infants still sleep prone and there has been little change in parental smoking habits. The justification for public health advice about other environmental risk factors should be kept under review. Excessive wrapping should be discouraged in older babies who are unwell, although there may be dangers in recommendations which increase the proportion of infants who are lightly wrapped.[59,90,91] Further evidence is required before recommendations can be made about breast-feeding and bed sharing.[92]

KEY POINTS FOR CLINICAL PRACTICE

- On average, SIDS affects less than 1 in 1200 infants but is still a major cause of death in infants after 1 month of age.
- The likelihood of finding an explanation for death in infants who die suddenly and unexpectedly has increased as the incidence of SIDS has fallen; such deaths should be thoroughly investigated.

To reduce the risk of SIDS:

- Avoid the prone sleeping position after the first month of life.
- Mothers should avoid smoking during and after pregnancy.
- There is no conclusive evidence that bed sharing increases the risk of SIDS.
- There is some evidence to suggest that excessive wrapping, particularly if the baby is unwell, may increase the risk of SIDS.

REFERENCES

1 Office of Population Censuses and Surveys. Sudden infant deaths 1988 to 1992. OPCS Monit 1993; DH3 93/2
2 Office of Population Censuses and Surveys. Sudden infant deaths 1985–87 OPCS Monit 1988; DH3 88/3
3 Registrar General Scotland. Annual report 1992. Edinburgh: General Register Office for Scotland, 1993; 138
4 Mitchell EA, Tonkin S. Publicity and infant's sleeping position. Br Med J 1993; 306: 858
5 Beal S. Sudden infant death syndrome related to sleeping position and bedding. Med J Aust 1991; 155: 507–508
6 De Jonge GA, Burgmeijer RJF, Engelberts AC, Hoogenboezem J, Kostense PJ, Sprij AJ. Sleeping position for infants and cot death in The Netherlands 1985–1991. Arch Dis Child 1993; 69: 660–663
7 Markestad T, Irgens LM, Baste V, Oyen N, Schreuder P. Infants' sleeping position and SIDS in Norway, 1970–1991. In: Proceedings of The European Society for the Study and Prevention of Infant Deaths (Third Congress). Oxford: 1993; Abstract 46
8 Helweg-Larsen K, Bille J, Iversen L. SIDS in Denmark, recent trends. A survey of a national campaign 'Back to Sleep'. In: Proceedings of The European Society for the Study and Prevention of Infant Deaths (Third Congress). Oxford: 1993; Abstract 42
9 Kiberd B. Ireland's first national sudden infant death register. Interim report 1992. In: Proceedings of The European Society for the Study and Prevention of Infant Deaths (Third Congress). Oxford: 1993; Abstract 38
10 Gilbert R. The changing epidemiology of SIDS. Arch Dis Child 1994; 70: 445–449
11 Frogatt P. In: Bergman AB, Beckwith JB, Ray GC, eds. Sudden infant death syndrome.

Seattle: University of Washington Press, 1970

12 Beal S. Sleeping position and sudden infant death syndrome. Med J Aust 1988; 149: 562

13 Tonkin SL. Infant mortality: epidemiology of cot deaths in Auckland. NZ Med J 1986; 99: 324–326

14 Beal SM, Finch CF. An overview of retrospective case-control studies investigating the relationship between prone sleeping position and SIDS J Paediatr Child Health 1991; 27: 334–339

15 Nicholl JP, O'Cathain A. Sleeping position and SIDS [Letter]. Lancet 1988; 2: 106

16 Kahn A, Blum D, Hennart P et al. A critical comparison of the history of sudden death infants and infants hospitalised for near-miss SIDS. Eur J Pediatr 1984; 143: 103–107

17 Cameron MH, Williams AL. Development and testing of scoring systems for predicting infants with high-risk of sudden infant death syndrome in Melbourne. Aust Paediatr J 1986; 22 (suppl): 37–45

18 Senecal J, Roussey M, Defawe G, Delahaye M, Piquemal B. Procubitus et mort subite inattendue du nourrisson. Arch Fr Pediatr 1987; 44: 131–136

19 Lee NNY, Chan YF, Davies DP, Lau E, Yip DCP. Sudden infant death syndrome in Hong Kong: confirmation of low incidence. Br Med J 1989; 298: 721

20 McGlashan ND. Sleeping position and SIDS [Letter]. Lancet 1988; 2: 106

21 De Jonge GA, Engelberts AC, Koomen-Liefting AJM, Kostense PJ. Cot death and prone sleeping position in The Netherlands. Br Med J 1989; 298: 722

22 Dwyer T, Ponsonby ALB, Newman NM, Gibbons LE. Prospective cohort study of prone sleeping position and sudden infant death syndrome. Lancet 1991; 337: 1244–1247

23 Mitchell EA, Scragg R, Stewart AW et al. Results from the first year of the New Zealand cot death study. NZ Med J 1991; 104(906): 71–76

24 Engelberts AC. Cot death in the Netherlands. An epidemiological study [Thesis]. Amsterdam: VU University Press, 1991

25 Fleming PJ, Gilbert RE, Azaz Y et al. Interaction between SID victims bedding and sleeping position in the sudden infant death syndrome: a population based case-control study. Br Med J 1990; 301: 85–89

26 Wigfield RE, Fleming PJ, Berry PJ, Rudd PT, Golding J. Can the fall in Avon's sudden infant death rate be explained by changes in sleeping position? Br Med J 1992; 304: 282–283

27 Gibbons LE, Ponsonby AL, Dwyer T. A comparison of prospective and retrospective responses on sudden infant death syndrome by case and control mothers. Am J Epidemiol 1993; 137: 654–659

28 Guntheroth WG, Spiers PS. Sleeping prone and the risk of sudden infant death syndrome. JAMA 1992; 267: 2359–2362

29 Department of Health. Report of the Chief Medical Officer's Expert Group on the sleeping position of infants and cot death. London: HMSO, 1993

30 Nelson EAS, Taylor BJ, Weatherall IL. Sleeping position and infant bedding may predispose to hyperthermia and the sudden infant death syndrome. Lancet 1989; 1: 199–201

31 Tonkin SL. Sudden infant death syndrome; a hypothesis of causation. Pediatrics 1975; 55: 650–661

32 Mitchell EA, Engelberts AC. Sleeping position and cot deaths [Letter]. Lancet 1991; 338: 192

33 Mitchell EA, Taylor BJ, Ford RPK et al. Dummies and the sudden infant death syndrome. Arch Dis Child 1993; 68: 501–504

34 Howat WJ, Moore IE, Judd M, Roche WR. Pulmonary immunopathology of sudden infant death syndrome. Lancet 1994; 343: 1390

35 Morris JA. Hypothesis: common bacterial toxins are a possible cause of the sudden infant death syndrome. Med Hypotheses 1987; 22: 211–222

36 Martinez FD. Sudden infant death syndrome and small airway occlusion: facts and a hypothesis. Pediatrics 1991: 87: 190–198

37 Blumenthal I, Lealman GT. Effect of posture on gastro-oesophageal reflux in the newborn. Arch Dis Child 1982; 57: 555–556

38 Beal S, Porter C. Sudden infant death syndrome related to climate. Acta Paediatr Scand 1991; 80: 278–287

39 Engelberts AC, De Jonge GA, Kostense PJ. An analysis of trends in the incidence of

sudden infant death in The Netherlands 1969–89. J Paediatr Child Health 1991; 27: 329–333

40 Mitchell EA, Ford RPK, Taylor BJ et al. Further evidence supporting a causal relationship between prone sleeping position and SIDS. J Paediatr Child Health 1992: 28 (suppl 1): S9–12

41 Fleming PJ. Personal communication 1993

42 Masterson J, Zucker C, Schulze K. Prone and supine positioning effects on energy expenditure and behaviour of low birth weight neonates. Pediatrics 1987; 80: 689–691

43 Hiley C. Babies' sleeping position [Letter]. Br Med J 1992; 305: 115

44 Mitchell EA, Aley P, Eastwood J. The national cot death prevention program in New Zealand. Aust J Public Health 1992; 16: 158–161

45 American Academy of Pediatrics Task Force on Infant Positioning and SIDS. Positioning and SIDS. Pediatrics 1992; 89: 1120–1126

46 Gibson AAM. Current epidemiology of SIDS. J Clin Pathol 1992; 45 (suppl): 7–10

47 Gilbert RE. The role of infection in sudden unexpected infant death [MD thesis]. University of Sheffield, 1993

48 Rintahaka PJ, Hirvonen J. The epidemiology of sudden infant death syndrome in Finland in 1969–1980. Forensic Sci Int 1986; 30: 219–233

49 Bulterys MG, Greenland S, Kraus JF. Chronic fetal hypoxia and sudden infant death syndrome: interaction between maternal smoking and low hematocrit during pregnancy. Pediatrics 1990; 86: 535–540

50 Haglund B, Cnattingius S. Cigarette smoking as a risk factor for sudden infant death syndrome: a population based study. Am J Public Health 1990: 80: 29–32

51 Weirenga H, Brand R, Geudeke T et al. Prenatal risk factors for cot death in very preterm and small for gestational age infants. Early Hum Dev 1990; 23: 15–26

52 Hoffman HJ, Damus K, Hillman L, Krongrad E. Risk factors for SIDS. Results of the National Institute of Child Health and Human Development SIDS cooperative epidemiological study. In: Schwartz PJ, Southall DP, Valdes-Dapena M, eds. The sudden infant death syndrome. Cardiac and respiratory mechanisms and interventions. Ann N Y Acad Sci 1988; 533: 13–30

53 Nicholl JP, O'Cathain A. Antenatal smoking, postnatal passive smoking and the sudden infant death syndrome. In: Poswillo D, Alberman E, eds. Effects of smoking on the fetus, neonate and child. Oxford: Oxford University Press, 1992: 138–149

54 Malloy MH, Kleinman JC, Land GH, Schramm WF. The association of maternal smoking with age and cause of infant deaths. Am J Epidemiol 1988; 128: 46–55

55 Murphy FJ, Newcombe RG, Sibert JR. The epidemiology of sudden infant death syndrome. J Epidemiol Community Health 1982; 36: 17–21

56 Bergman AB, Wiesner LA. Relationship of passive cigarette smoking to sudden infant death syndrome. Pediatrics 1976; 58: 665–668

57 McGlashan ND. Sudden infant deaths in Tasmania, 1980–1986: a seven year prospective study. Soc Sci Med 1989; 29: 1015–1026

58 Fleming KA. Viral respiratory infection and SIDS. J Clin Pathol 1992; 45 (suppl): 29–32

59 Gilbert RE, Rudd PT, Berry PJ et al. Combined effect of infection and heavy wrapping on the risk of sudden unexpected infant death. Arch Dis Child 1992; 67: 171–177

60 Urquhart GED, Grist NR. Virological studies of sudden, unexplained infant deaths in Glasgow 1967–70. J Clin Pathol 1972; 25: 443–446

61 Ray CG, Beckwith JB, Hebestreit NM, Bergman AB. Studies of the sudden infant death syndrome in King County, Washington. The role of viruses. JAMA 1970; 211: 619–623

62 Williams AL, Uren EC, Bretherton L. Respiratory viruses and sudden infant death. Br Med J 1984; 288: 1491–1493

63 Carpenter RG, Shaddick CW. Role of infection, suffocation and bottle feeding in cot death. An analysis of some factors in the histories of 110 cases and their controls. Br J Prev Soc Med 1965; 19: 1–7

64 Protestos CD, Carpenter RG, McWeeny PM, Emery JL. Obstetric and perinatal histories of children who died unexpectedly (cot death). Arch Dis Child 1973; 48: 835–841

65 Biering-Sorensen F, Jorgensen T, Hilden J. Sudden infant death in Copenhagen. Acta Paediatr Scand 1978; 67: 129–137

66 Watson E, Gardner A, Carpenter RG. An epidemiological and sociological study of unexpected death in infancy in nine areas of Southern England. Med Sci Law 1981; 21: 78–98

67 Harris JDC, Radford M, Wailoo M, Carpenter RG, Machin K. Sudden infant death in Southampton and an evaluation of the Sheffield scoring system. J Epidemiol Community Health 1982; 36: 162–166

68 Knowelden J, Keeling J, Nicholl JP. A multicentre study of postneonatal mortality. London: HMSO, 1984

69 Beal SM. Sudden infant death syndrome: epidemiological comparisons between South Australia and communities with a different incidence. Aust Paediatr J 1986; 22: 13–16

70 Ford RPK, Taylor BJ, Mitchell EA et al. Breastfeeding and the risk of sudden infant death syndrome. Int J Epidemiol 1993; 22: 885–889

71 Frogatt P, Lynas MA, MacKenzie G. Epidemiology of sudden unexpected death in infants (cot death) in Northern Ireland. Br J Prev Soc Med 1971; 49: 119–134

72 Kraus AS, Steele R, Thompson MG, de Grosbois P. Further epidemiologic observations on sudden death in infancy in Ontario. Can J Public Health 1971; 62: 210–218

73 Rhead WJ, Schrauzer GN, Saltstein SL. Sudden death in infancy and vitamin E deficiency [Letter]. Br Med J 1973; 4: 548–549

74 Fedrick J. Sudden unexpected death in infants in the Oxford Record Linkage Area. Br J Prev Soc Med 1974; 28: 164–171

75 Kraus JF, Greenland S, Bulterys M. Risk factors for sudden infant death in the US collaborative perinatal project. Int J Epidemiol 1989; 18: 113–120

76 Ponsonby AL, Dwyer T, Gibbons LE, Cochrane JA, Jones ME, McCall MJ. Thermal environment and sudden infant death syndrome: case-control study. Br Med J 1992; 304: 277–282

77 Wigfield RE. Personal communication 1993

78 Petersen SA, Anderson ES, Lodemore M, Rawson D, Wailoo MP. Sleeping position and rectal temperature. Arch Dis Child 1991; 66: 976–979

79 McKenna JJ, Thoman EB, Anders TF, Schechtman VL, Glotzbach SF. Infant–parent co-sleeping in an evolutionary perspective: implications for understanding infant sleep development and the sudden infant death syndrome. Sleep 1993; 16: 63–82

80 Scragg R, Mitchell EA, Taylor BJ et al. Bed sharing, smoking and alcohol in the sudden infant death syndrome. Br Med J 1993; 307: 1312–1318

81 Tuohy PG, Counsell AM, Geddis DC. Sociodemographic factors associated with sleeping position and location. Arch Dis Child 1993; 69: 664–666

82 Phillips AN, Smith GD. How independent are 'independent' effects? Relative risk estimation when correlated exposures are measured imprecisely. J Clin Epidemiol 1991; 44: 1223–1231

83 Hoffman HJ. Personal communication 1993

84 Mitchell EA. International trends in postneonatal mortality. Arch Dis Child 1990; 65: 607–609

85 Brooke H, Gibson AAM, The Scottish Cot Death Trust. Personal communication 1993

86 Lee M, Davies DP, Chan YF. Prone or supine for preterm babies [Letter]. Lancet 1988; 1: 1332

87 Scott A, Campbell H, Gorman D. Sudden infant death syndrome in Scotland. Br Med J 1993; 306: 211–212

88 Madeley RJ, Hull D, Holland T. Prevention of postneonatal mortality. Arch Dis Child 1986; 61: 459–463

89 White A, Nicholaas G, Foster K, Browne F, Carey S. Health survey for England, 1991. London: Office of Population Censuses and Surveys, 1993

90 Wigfield RE, Fleming PJ, Howell T et al. How much wrapping do babies need at night? Arch Dis Child 1993; 69: 181–186

91 Dunne KP, Matthews TG. Hypothermia and SIDS. Arch Dis Child 1988; 63: 438–440

92 Health Education Authority. New pregnancy book. London: The Health Education Authority, 1993

4. Current thoughts on hearing screening

A. Davis

Hearing screening is a major health care activity in early childhood. It is important to understand why it is undertaken, how effective the set of current hearing screening activities have been and the way in which these activities should change over the next few years to produce a more cost-effective service. In this chapter I hope to provide some answers to these questions, by exploring the health care context in which hearing screening takes place, the epidemiology of hearing impairment in young children in the present generation, the developments in the methods of screening that have taken place over the last decade and the impact that well-targeted and well-formulated information technology might have on the organization of services.

The gearing of hearing screening service provision towards those services that have been appropriately evaluated, instantiated effectively and properly audited is something that is urgently required by purchasers and providers. However, there is confusion about how best to implement hearing screening in a 'typical' health district. At present, there is considerable heterogeneity in the services that different districts provide, and in the success of those services. It is possible that some districts still do not know how well, or how badly, they are performing and there is no policy with respect to attaining the appropriate 'intelligence' about service performance as a whole. Poor records systems are a major barrier in managing hearing health care.[1] In particular, hearing screening needs effective information systems to work well. The absence of these systems inevitably leads to poor management of individual children and poorly tuned services for all hearing impaired children.

On the other hand, well-run screening services, in conjunction with an integrated information system, can facilitate not only the management of individual children but also the management of the hearing health care programme as a whole. In a well-run service the coverage rates, onward referral rates, incremental yields and appropriate outcome measures are indicators that enable purchasers with a knowledge of the local epidemiology of hearing impairments to make decisions about how the services should be funded and developed. Without these data it is quite difficult!

There are a considerable number of different providers and professional groups involved both in hearing screening and in the provision of rehabilitative services, e.g. paediatricians, health visitors, neonatal nurses, neonatologists, audiologists, medical physicists, otologists, audiological physicians, educators, hearing therapists, speech therapists, social workers, voluntary organizations and community paediatricians. It is precisely because of the interdisciplinary nature of hearing screening and rehabilitation that it can and does fall between the responsibilities of one group or another. There is a prima facie case that an individual (e.g. chair of the audiology working party) in each district should be identified who has the responsibility for the hearing screening programme as a whole.[2] In the present National Health Service (NHS) reorganization this may not be possible, but it would certainly go some way towards improving the present services and creating a seamless service that is much more user-friendly than those presently provided.

In the following sections, I will concentrate on the three key questions posed above. The descriptive epidemiology of hearing impairments will shed light on the question, why is hearing screening undertaken? However, the second question is less easy to answer: what do the present set of services achieve? I know from personal experience how hearing screening operates in a number of districts. A common feature appears to be that no-one is particularly satisfied with their set-up and that advice on how to set up better services is widely sought.

One of the problems with reviewing present services is that there are no national data collected with respect to either the organization of the services themselves or of the services provided for hearing impaired children. If there was a national register of permanently hearing impaired children, for instance, then it would be easier to assess some of the appropriate process data, such as age of identification, age of hearing aid fitting, false positive rate, cost and, most importantly, false negatives. In addition to these data, appropriately stratified, such a register might facilitate (1) the formation of more optimal service models, (2) the formulation of better preventive strategies through a more detailed national epidemiology of permanent childhood hearing impairment, (3) research into the outcomes achieved by hearing impaired children and the factors that are related to 'better' outcomes. For reasons that will become obvious in the epidemiology section, it is meaningless to look at the cost-utility or cost-effectiveness of hearing and rehabilitative services in individual districts over a short period of time; such audit can only be conducted over a long time span or over a wide area.

However, it is easy to see where systems are not working. For example, in many districts it is not possible to find out the coverage rate of the Health Visitor Distraction Test (HVDT); in others no hearing impaired child has been detected by the HVDT for 4 or 5 years, while in others referral rates from hearing screening are inducing very long delays (>9 months) in the assessment system thus delaying treatment for those who are hearing impaired.

Whilst there are signs that the hearing screening systems in the UK need some reorganization and possible standardization, the UK is probably ahead of countries such as the USA and much of central and southern Europe in terms of age of detection of permanently hearing impaired children. The problem is that, except in some exceptional districts, it does not meet a 'simple goal'[3,4] such as detecting all congenitally hearing impaired children by the age of 6 months. The next section looks at this comparative context for hearing screening.

BACKGROUND AND CONTEXT

The major comparative context in which hearing screening is currently debated is the consensus statement issued by the US National Institutes of Health (NIH).[5] This document emphasizes the fact that the lack of early detection of hearing impaired chiildren is a major public health problem and endorses the aim outlined above to detect congenital hearing impairment by the age of 6 months. The task of detection for those with a moderate, severe or profound bilateral hearing impairment is divided into three populations: (1) those 7–10% of births at high risk (babies in neonatal intensive care units (NICU) or well babies with either craniofacial abnormalities, a family history of hearing impairment, or intrauterine infections), (2) the remainder of births, and (3) those children who have late-acquired hearing impairments (predominantly meningitis).

Among the NIH documents, there is very little evidence that early detection is better for all degrees and types of hearing impairment, and this is an area where further research is needed to clarify exactly what benefit, and to whom, very early detection confers. The NIH consensus takes this for granted and suggests that the major areas that benefit are language, speech and emotional/social development. Leaving this aside for now, in the subtext of the statement three recommendations are made for each of the three populations. First, at 'small cost' the high-risk children should be screened before leaving hospital care. Second, at much greater cost, consideration should be given to introducing well-baby screening. Third, every child who has meningitis should be referred for a hearing test.

Dealing with this last item first, the recommendation was to screen/test the child prior to discharge. In the UK, we have found that this is not an optimum time due to the difficulty of testing children of this age and also the very large proportion of children who have a conductive hearing pathology.[6–8] We suggested that, whilst concerns of severe/profound hearing impairment should always be acted upon as soon as possible, an appointment for a thorough hearing assessment should be made prior to discharge and for a time some 4–6 weeks post discharge. The larger distances in the USA and the greater numbers of children who may come from areas with relatively poor childhood health care provision might militate against this scheme, but almost certainly sedation for auditory brainstem response (ABR) testing might have to be used if a total coverage of this population were to be made prior to discharge.

In the conclusions of the NIH consensus statement little distinction is made between the first two populations. The recommendations were that a first screen should be carried out, as close to discharge of the baby as possible, using otoacoustic emissions, and if the baby did not pass this first screen a second screen using ABR should be used to cut down on the number of false positives (up to 10%) from the first screen. In failing to carry through in its entirety the previous distinction between the two populations the consensus statement[5] has recommended that, 'because of the unique accessibility of almost all infants in the newborn nursery, the consensus panel recommends screening for *all* newborns, both high and low risk, for hearing impairment prior to hospital discharge' (p 19).

This ideal recommendation has caused a considerable increase in hearing screening activity in the USA, and an increase in related research. However, there is doubt as to whether the flurry of activity is the best way to proceed and whether all the preconditions and principles for screening[9–13] are met within the USA context. There is no guidance given on how the transition from present arrangements to universal screening may be achieved (or financed). From the UK perspective there must be considerable doubt as to whether this is the best way to proceed with our population and in the context of the UK health care system.[14]

Two sets of recommendations exist in the UK at present. The report on the Joint Working Party on Child Health Surveillance[2,15] has a set of recommendations that stems from a systematic review of the literature and some information concerning current practice. This endorses the need to have a systematic approach to raising parental awareness through check-lists (which are often made available through parent-held child health records) of hearing impairment and disability at all stages of development and for professionals to act when concern is voiced by parents. In addition, formal use of screening methods such as the HVDT and school screening are recommended. The UK context and tradition is substantially different to that in the USA[11] in having, in principle, these two occasions when every child is screened for hearing impairment. The report is more tentative concerning neonatal screening, and suggests that it should be regarded as 'in a research phase'.

However, the more recent National Deaf Children's Society (NDCS) quality standards for the early identification of children with hearing impairments goes further than this in its recommendations.[16] These standards were drawn up by a group of 'experts' addressing a specific problem, i.e. the identification of bilateral moderate and (worse) permanently hearing impaired children. The documents were sent to all relevant professional societies for comment prior to publication. So the status of the standards is not one of thoroughly tried and evaluated guidelines, more a stimulus for action and debate as well as an expression of concern for present practice.

The targets recommended by the NDCS document[16] differed from the aims endorsed by the NIH consensus from the Joint Committee on Infant Hearing (JCIH) and mentioned above as 'to identify and begin treatment for all hearing impaired children by 6 months of age'. Such a target was seen as too extreme for districts to achieve over the next 5 years. Thus the first target set was 'to detect 80% of bilateral congenital hearing impairments in excess of 50 dB HL . . . within the first year of life and 40% by the age of six months' (para 2.1). Two further targets related to the provision of hearing aids and provision of tests for those at risk of acquired hearing impairment.[7,8] The fourth target was 'to ensure that by 1 year of age *all* children resident in a district will have benefited from either a formal screen or a specific surveillance procedure to see if they are at risk of hearing loss' (para 2.4).

The minimum requirements for a good quality service and for documenting the targets are set out in detail. The underlying sentiment is that 'targeted neonatal screening and improved child health surveillance procedures need to be introduced as a matter of priority. The alternative approach of universal neonatal screening should be given careful thought and consideration for the future' (para 3).

The public health task, therefore, is made explicit in terms of the transitions from present arrangements that need to occur. First, introduce targeted neonatal screening as a matter of some urgency, if not already implemented. Second, tighten up on the child health surveillance procedures, including (1) the HVDT if it has been retained and (2) provision of adequate information on the present services. Third, when appropriate and well evaluated, consider the introduction of universal neonatal screening together with revised targets for age of detection.

The protocol for targeted neonatal screening and for non-high-risk children is laid out in some detail, but the document pulls back from exclusively recommending any particular method for neonatal or the 6–7–month screening. This is sensible because at present there are no wholly convincing data that any one method gives substantially better results; rather, the evidence indicates that sites with commitments to particular methods do better with those methods. This suggests that there is still a need for appropriate post-implementation evaluations that look at the factors that predispose to more consistent results. The major problem is that, unless a more coordinated national approach to implementation is taken rather than on a district to district basis, it is very difficult to identify those factors!

When should universal neonatal screening be considered in the future? It would probably cost a minimum of £8–10 million to introduce neonatal screening in all health districts and health boards in the UK, in terms of direct staffing costs (£10–12 per child screened), to obtain 90% coverage rate (this is similar to the staffing requirement deduced by Hunter et al.[17]). However, other costs would probably increase this per capita figure. As well as considering the cost-effectiveness of the universal neonatal screening procedures, a decision would also have to be made about whether to retain the

HVDT. It may not be possible to phase one out and the other in overnight, especially as the value of doing the HVDT (or the neonatal screen) may not only include its face valid component. For instance, the HVDT may have an added function in detecting those children most at risk of having persistent 'glue ear'. In an ideal world the incremental yield for permanent childhood hearing impairment of the HVDT would be monitored after the introduction of neonatal screening together with any other benefits thought relevant before phasing it out. This argues for a more complex financing of universal screening than a straight swop for the HVDT.

At present, however, despite encouraging reports from sites in the USA,[18] it is premature to embark upon isolated service programmes of universal neonatal screening. The scope for limited post-implementation evaluations is clear and there are now experimental programmes of universal screening using transient evoked otoacoustic emissions (TEOAE) in the UK.[17,19] The trial of neonatal screening being conducted in the Wessex and South West Regions of the NHS by Kennedy and his colleagues may give a good idea of its effectiveness by the end of 1995. At the same time the results of a systematic review of hearing screening, with particular reference to the role of neonatal screening, commissioned by the Department of Health should also be available.

At present, districts should plan to introduce targeted neonatal screening, review the efficacy of their HVDT programme and prime purchasers concerning the direction in which services might evolve over the next few years. Proposals for universal neonatal hearing screening have a long history.[20,21] To be worthwhile, programmes need to have high sensitivity and good cost-effectiveness, to be applicable for high-risk as well as non-high-risk infants, and in the long term to show better outcomes. It is not clear to me that at present we know that this is the case.

EPIDEMIOLOGY OF PERMANENT CHILDHOOD HEARING IMPAIRMENT

How many children are hearing impaired?

A comparison of a number of different studies on the incidence or annual birth cohort prevalence of permanent childhood hearing impairment is given in Davis,[1] Mauk & Behrens[22] and Davidson et al.[23] The incidence depends on the severity of the hearing impairment, the definition of a 'case', all well as on how well all 'cases' were ascertained. For the UK, the work of Davis & Wood,[24] Davis et al[25] and Davis & Parving[26] suggests an incidence of congenital permanent bilateral hearing impairment, per 100 000 birth cohort, of 116 (confidence interval (CI) 102–131) for children with bilateral hearing impairments of ≥ 40 dB HL (hearing level). For the present birth cohort (about 780 000) in the UK, this is about 900 children and by the age of 5 years we might expect about another 80–90 children with late-acquired hearing impairments. By the age of 5 years the birth cohort prevalence, from all causes, is 41 per 100 000 (CI 33–51) for ≥95 dB HL and about 27 for ≥105 dB HL, which is the level at which cochlear implantation candidature is currently operating.[27] This would suggest somewhere in the region of 240 children per birth cohort are potential candidates for cochlear implants, using current criteria.

Table 4.1 gives estimates for the number of hearing impaired children in England and Wales as a function of country, county, age group and severity of hearing impairment. The population data on which they are based is the OPCS (Office of Population Censuses and Surveys) mid-1992 estimates of resident population in England and Wales for 5-year age groups (and under 1 year of age). The counts for the age groups shown in Table 4.1 were derived by interpolation of the OPCS data. To derive the number of children in each severity band the data of Davis & Parving[26] were used for the two ranges of hearing impairment (≥40 dB HL and ≥95 dB HL). Care must be taken in interpreting the table in three ways: (1) the ≥95 dB HL data are included in the ≥40 dB HL data, so do not add them together, (2) the under 1-year-olds are also included in the ≤4 years data, so do not add these data together, and (3) these are estimates derived from several local studies[26] and do not represent the actual number of children with hearing impairment in these districts. The actual number of children may be bigger, to reflect the better ascertainment in older age groups (which would not have been the case from our studies). In addition, the number of profoundly hearing impaired children may be larger, especially in the 12–18-year-olds where different aetiologies may account for a different pattern of severity than found in recent studies.[1,28] The best estimate of the number of hearing impaired children (≥40 dB HL) in England and Wales, from Table 4.1, is 14 296 (CI 12 573–16 146). In Table 4.1, the confidence intervals for the estimates are about ± 12% of the estimates. In terms of profoundly hearing impaired children there are probably somewhere in the region of 4000 to 5000 children of school age in England and Wales.

What are the major risk factors?

Many of the neonatal and high-risk screening programmes in the UK use a number of risk factors to define their target group. For children with a congenital hearing impairment in the UK the major risk factors are (1) NICU history accounting for 32% (CI 26–40), (2) a family history of congenital/early childhood hearing impairment accounting for 25% (CI 21–34) given no NICU history, and (3) abnormal craniofacial presentation, adding about 7% (given neither NICU or family history) to these prior two factors.[25] Taken together, these three risk factors account for about two-thirds (CI 57–72%) of the hearing impaired children in the UK, from data collected in the mid-1980s (it is not possible to include more recent data because of the

Table 4.1 The estimated number of hearing impaired children in England and Wales by County district and age group using the 1992 OPCS population estimates in two severity bands ≥40 dB HL and 95 dB HL

	All children (0–18 years)			Under 1 year		≤4 years		5–11 years		12–18 years	
	Count	≥40 dB*	≥95 dB	≥40 dB	≥95 dB	≥40 dB	≥95 dB	≥40 dB	≥95 dB	≥40 dB	≥95 dB
Country											
England and Wales	12325279	14296	4433	805	249	4006	1242	5230	1622	5058	1568
England	11618765	13476	4179	761	236	3784	1173	4926	1527	4765	1477
Wales	706513	819	254	43	13	222	69	304	94	292	90
County											
Greater London	1595411	1850	573	121	37	569	176	667	206	613	190
Greater Manchester	652966	757	234	43	13	216	67	279	86	261	81
Merseyside	362269	420	130	22	7	116	36	156	48	147	45
South Yorkshire	308241	357	110	20	6	101	31	130	40	125	39
Tyne and Wear	271779	315	97	17	5	86	26	116	36	112	34
West Midlands	670084	777	241	45	14	222	68	285	88	269	83
West Yorkshire	526278	610	189	34	10	172	53	223	69	214	66
Avon	223491	259	80	14	4	72	22	93	29	93	28
Bedfordshire	140327	162	50	9	2	46	14	59	18	56	17
Berkshire	189967	220	68	12	3	61	19	80	24	78	24
Buckinghamshire	167873	194	60	10	3	52	16	71	22	70	21
Cambridgeshire	166485	193	59	10	3	53	16	69	21	70	21
Cheshire	238072	276	85	14	4	75	23	102	31	98	30
Cleveland	148790	172	53	9	2	46	14	65	20	60	18
Cornwall and Scilly	108415	125	38	6	1	32	10	46	14	45	14
Cumbria	112966	131	40	7	2	35	10	48	14	47	14

Table 4.1 (Continued)

	All children (0–18 years)			Under 1 year		≤4 years		5–11 years		12–18 years	
	Count	≥40 dB*	≥95 dB	≥40 dB	≥95 dB	≥40 dB	≥95 dB	≥40 dB	≥95 dB	≥40 dB	≥95 dB
Derbyshire	223172	258	80	14	4	71	22	94	29	92	28
Devon	232751	269	83	14	4	72	22	98	30	99	30
Dorset	140792	163	50	8	2	43	13	59	18	60	18
Durham	145655	168	52	9	2	45	14	62	19	60	18
East Sussex	150965	175	54	9	2	49	15	64	19	61	19
Essex	372535	432	134	23	7	119	37	156	48	155	48
Gloucestershire	126846	147	45	7	2	40	12	53	16	52	16
Hampshire	379521	440	136	24	7	123	38	160	49	156	48
Hereford and Worcester	166198	192	59	10	3	51	15	70	21	70	21
Hertfordshire	240540	279	86	15	4	78	24	101	31	99	30
Humberside	218170	253	78	13	4	69	21	93	28	90	27
Isle of Wight	27272	31	9	1	0	7	2	11	3	11	3
Kent	373560	433	134	23	7	119	37	157	48	156	48
Lancashire	348416	404	125	22	6	111	34	149	46	143	44
Leicestershire	226460	262	81	14	4	72	22	95	29	94	29
Lincolnshire	136584	158	49	8	2	41	12	58	18	58	18
Norfolk	170157	197	61	10	3	52	16	71	22	73	22
Northamptonshire	151417	175	54	9	2	48	15	64	20	62	19
Northumberland	72707	84	26	4	1	21	6	31	9	31	9
North Yorkshire	163670	189	58	9	3	50	15	69	21	70	21
Nottinghamshire	245893	285	88	16	4	79	24	103	32	101	31
Oxfordshire	143878	166	51	9	2	46	14	59	18	60	18

Table 4.1 (Continued)

	All children (0–18 years)			Under 1 year		≤4 years		5–11 years		12–18 years	
	Count	≥40 dB*	≥95 dB	≥40 dB	≥95 dB	≥40 dB	≥95 dB	≥40 dB	≥95 dB	≥40 dB	≥95 dB
Shropshire	101754	118	36	6	1	31	9	43	13	43	13
Somerset	111537	129	40	6	2	34	10	46	14	48	14
Staffordshire	255269	296	91	15	4	81	25	109	33	105	32
Suffolk	157066	182	56	9	3	50	15	66	20	65	20
Surrey	237241	275	85	14	4	74	23	99	30	101	31
Warwickshire	116171	134	41	6	2	36	11	49	15	49	15
West sussex	158025	183	56	9	3	49	15	67	20	66	20
Wiltshire	141109	163	50	8	2	46	14	59	18	57	17
Clwyd	99746	115	35	6	1	30	9	42	13	42	13
Dyfed	82013	95	29	4	1	24	7	35	11	35	10
Gwent	111646	129	40	7	2	36	11	48	14	44	13
Gwynedd	55905	64	20	3	1	17	5	23	7	24	7
Mid Glamorgan	138481	160	49	8	2	44	13	60	18	56	17
Powys	27555	31	9	1	0	8	2	11	3	11	3
South Glamorgan	102573	118	36	6	2	33	10	43	13	41	12
West Glamorgan	88591	102	31	5	1	27	8	38	11	37	11

* Hearing level.

Care must be taken in interpreting the table in three ways: (1) the ≥95 dB HL data are included in the ≥40 dB HL data, so do not add them together, (2) the under 1-year-olds are also included in the ≤4 years data, so do not add these data together, and (3) these are estimates derived from several local studies[26] and do not represent the actual number of children with hearing impairment in these districts.

problems in ascertainment). Vanniasegaram et al[29] have suggested that ethnic origin may also be a risk factor in some inner city populations.

This pattern of the major three risk factors does not appear to be culturally/geographically independent. Whilst within the UK samples there was no gross difference in the ratio between the three factors, there was a substantial difference between the Danish data and that from the UK.[26] This shows that the proportion of hearing impaired children with a NICU history in the UK was about twice that of Denmark, and conversely the proportion with a family history of congenital hearing impairments in Denmark was twice that in the UK. This latter finding was ascribed, in part, to the larger proportion of consanguinous marriages in Denmark among the different ethnic minorities. However, there did not appear to be any explanation for the difference between the contribution of the NICU history children in the two countries.

It does appear, therefore, in the UK that if a screening programme effectively uses these three risk factors then it could find almost two-thirds of hearing impaired children. If the yield of the children with a family history is only half of that expected, then about 50% should be possible. However, if there are substantial variations in local epidemiology of hearing impairment then these data may be misleading. Hence it is important to try to understand the local epidemiology in a systematic way, for example by using an information system, such as a child health database, a register of children's disabilities, or a specific database such as the Paediatric Audiology Record System (PARS).[30] A minimum dataset for use with screening and in assessing local epidemiology is suggested in the NDCS paediatric audiology quality standards vol 1.[16]

Year on year the variation in the number of children in different risk categories may be quite large, as the Poisson distribution would suggest. It may also be the case that a routine service providing at risk screening, using NICU criteria and family history and craniofacial abnormality, may fall far short of the theoretical maximum; for example, it may give 30% rather than 60% due to coverage problems rather than sensitivity.

Such a gain, however, is achievable now and may be considered to be a vital first step in lowering the age of intervention in a group of children who are not only at risk for hearing impairment but also for cognitive sequelae. It may be more essential for these children that they are unencumbered by even mild to moderate auditory deprivation as the cortical development in such children may be more fragile than in non-NICU children. Additional information about the aetiologies that have been found in the UK is shown in Davis.[1]

What is the current age of identification of hearing impaired children?

It is a difficult task to find the distribution of the current age of identification of hearing impaired children. This is reliant even more on the completeness of ascertainment than the prevalence estimates. The tendency is to underestimate the true mean or median of the distribution, and hence the earlier you look the better the results tend to appear. To some extent the most appropriate statistics to consider are the percentiles of the distribution of the age of identification. The most commonly used percentiles are the median and the quartiles. So in England, over the years in the early to mid-1980s, the median age of identification, taken from the age at first appointment, was 12 months for the Nottingham and Sheffield districts and the Oxford region combined. The lower quartile was 8 months and the upper quartile 25 months.[25] In other words, over a quarter of the children with moderate ($\geq$40 dB HL) or worse hearing impairment were not identified until over 2 years of age! These data may be a somewhat optimistic estimate for the UK as a whole, for which no data are available in this format.

Data concerning the age of identification are not symmetrical about the mean or median. The distribution has a long tail and hence the mean age of identification is not near the median of 12 months, but 17 months.[25] The mean is thus very dependent on the late-detected cases and is very variable. However, the advantage of the mean is that it does show these outliers, and it really depends what weight is put on a child that is found at say 5 years compared to say 8 months. A lot depends on the severity of the hearing impairment how seriously one might weight a particular case. Ideally a weighted metric of age of identification is needed that takes the age and impairment of the child into account. To construct such a scale, however, needs an appropriate outcome study, which does not exist. However, for the present it is worth focusing on the percentiles of the distribution and the mean when judging how well particular systems of screening work. The NDCS quality standards (vol 1) suggest as a target that the 80th percentile of the age of detection for congenital hearing impaired children with better ear thresholds in mid-frequency $\geq$50 dB HL should be 12 months or less. This is half the 25 months of the upper quartile for the above study, and thus much work will be needed to achieve this target.

METHODS OF SCREENING CHILDREN'S HEARING

I do not intend to cover all the test methods for screening children's hearing. A standard text such as 'Paediatric audiology 0–5 years'[31] should be consulted to give the background to tests that are appropriate for particular ages of child. To some extent, I have found that there is a tendency to focus far too much on the test that is used, rather than on the other aspects of organizing a screening programme. The technology is enabling, but there is no need to let the technology dictate what should be done. The test is just one aspect of the screening programme and considerable attention should also be given to the aims of the programme, which children are tested, who carries out the test, what protocol is used for screen passes and fails, how results of the programme are monitored, what is the management structure of the programme, what audiological facilities are available, how parents are told the result of the test as well as what test equipment should be used.

Neonatal period

In the neonatal period there are currently three methods that one might consider: TEOAE, ABR and behavioural methods.

Otoacoustic emissions

Kemp[32] discovered that it is possible to measure with a tiny microphone the synchronized active process of a healthy cochlea when it is stimulated by a succession of clicks. Successful scientific, technological and commercial development of this has lead to the two machines being available to measure the TEOAE: the ILO88 and the ILO92. There is no intrinsic difference between the two machines, except that the ILO92 can carry out distortion product emissions and also other paradigms that are mainly of research interest at present.

One of the major potential uses of TEOAE is to screen for impaired hearing, particularly in those who cannot give a reliable verbal response. Hence there is considerable interest in the use of TEOAE for neonatal screening.

The NIH consensus statement recommended research on, development and use of TEOAE for universal screening because of its promise, non-invasiveness and the fact that it can potentially be carried out quite quickly (e.g. <10 min overall for a non-NICU baby, 36 h or more post delivery).

Experience will tell whether this is the right approach to mass screening and the role that it might have in targeted screening of those children at risk through NICU history. The European Union Concerted Action on Otoemission has set up a monitoring programme to look at the role of TEOAE in neonatal (and other childhood) hearing screening programmes. This sub-project, coordinated by Dr Adrian Davis, has agreed a common protocol and minimum dataset and will provide a preliminary report in December 1995. [*Note*: The protocol is available to anyone who requests it, together with an inspection copy of the accompanying PC database, from the author.]

Interest in applying the use of TEOAE as a universal screen has been considerable in the UK, and the result of the trials conducted by Dr Colin Kennedy and his colleagues is eagerly awaited in 1995. There has been some scepticism as to how extensive a coverage a neonatal screen can achieve in a modern hospital setting where the accent is on early discharge of well babies. In addition, there are practical problems because a much higher false positive rate is given in very young babies (less than 36 h than in older well babies). The mechanism for this is not known for certain and may be a mixture of fluid in the ear and/or oxygenation of the cochlea.[33]

We have conducted research with TEOAE in a multicentre study of their use for testing at-risk children. We used the IHR POEMS equipment,[34] which was designed for research purposes prior to the availability of the ILO88, as well as one of the first ILO88 machines. The major cause for concern with this ongoing study[35] was the high variability in screen failure rates between centres. The screen fail rate for the first test was averaging about 15–18% over the last 4 years. For the different sites the false positive rates were 14, 9, 26, 19, 33, 15, 17 and 8% with an overall of 18% ($N = 4298$ at-risk babies). There are considerable differences in the weight and gestational ages of the babies tested in different hospitals which accounts for much of the variation in false positive rates. NICU babies with birth weights under 1500 g had a false positive rate of 24% compared to the larger babies who had a false positive rate of 12% in the Nottingham NICUs ($N = 862$). In addition, some NICUs discharged babies back to referring hospitals at a much earlier stage than others. Such babies were often tested when no facilities for neonatal screen existed at the referring hospital. However, it is possible that the audiological management of the programmes might have a considerable influence on the outcomes. This is the case because no really effective automated algorithm for deciding on the presence/absence of an emission has yet been universally accepted. The pass/refer/retest decision is a real skill that has to be acquired by the person administering the test, and it should be monitored by a trained audiologist. The major strength of emissions is that it is highly sensitive to hearing impairment, even mild impairments.[34]

The usual protocol[5,17] is for children who fail a TEOAE to have a follow-up screen using ABR, rather than to be referred outright for a full audiological assessment.

Future developments of the TEOAE and other emission methods look very interesting and may overcome the current practical problems, such as probe fit in small neonates, high false positive rates in very young children and the theoretical problems concerning how to score the emissions. New technology may speed the measurement up or make it more robust so that a new generation of instruments may be hand-held and allow a measurement to be obtained within seconds rather than minutes. The potential is then expanded greatly and could, for example, be used in community-based screens.

Auditory brainstem responses

The use of ABR for determining hearing thresholds in children is well established and its development as a screening tool, particularly for at-risk children, has been researched over the last 12–14 years.[36] It takes more time than TEOAE and is more invasive. Electrodes, usually disposable ones, have to be attached to the neonate's head and the skin is usually mildly abraded. This is a small problem, but can be a nuisance if it disturbs the baby's sleep. Whilst very young there is no need for any sedation of the child.

Usually, children that fail a TEOAE screen have a follow-up screen with ABR. However, the main variable here is the level at which the ABR screen is carried out. The lower the level the higher the false positive rate. A reasonable compromise is 50 dB nHL, where the aim is to find those children with at least moderate to severe impairment. If used in tandem with the TEOAE this, of course, fixes a limit to the degree of hearing impairment that the TEOAE screen can find. In units where only a small number of at-risk babies are being tested, the ABR is really the most cost-effective method to use. The tester needs only one set of equipment and competency in ABR testing and assessment. However, in some ways the ABR does need a higher tester skill level than TEOAE.

In general, the gain from ABR screening, at say 50 dB nHL, is a lower level of false positives, which can be balanced against the extra time. Not only does this mean fewer re-screens, but also less parental anxiety. However, in the at-risk context, parental anxiety may be less of a problem than in the well-baby context where, at present, ABR is not a viable screening tool.

Behavioural methods

Behavioural methods have been used for quite a while as a possible screening test.[37] The Crib-o-Gram[38] and the Auditory Response Cradle[20,21] have both had limited trials in universal and at-risk contexts. For the at-risk neonatal population these methods are interesting, but probably not suitable. For the not-at-risk population there may be several advantages of the behavioural method, including its validity, time to test and false positive rate. However, its potential for future use is probably quite limited compared with the TEOAE. This is because the TEOAE is much more sensitive to moderate hearing impairments than the current generation of behavioural methods. So, only if we agree that the major priority is to find children with severe and profound hearing impairments at birth do behavioural methods enter the equation.

Screening at 6–8 months

There is general agreement[2,16] that the HVDT should be universally applied, providing that arrangements for its coverage, training and testing facilities meet high standards. The sensitivity of the HVDT can approach 90% for hearing impairments of >50 dB HL.[24] However, it is possible for this to dip well below 50% if coverage and levels of expertise are not maintained. When that is the case then one is giving false reassurance to an increasing number of parents. An alternative approach has been tried in Reading[39] using a more general surveillance approach without the HVDT. This needs considerable training as well, and relies more on a structured interview with the parents, especially eliciting any parental concerns vis-à-vis the child's communication and hearing. It is too early to see whether this works better than the HVDT.

It is worth pointing out that the Reading approach does not save on training or effort; however, it does only need one person and not two.

Future developments of behavioural testing can be expected. Particularly the use of microprocessors to generate the sound stimuli will become very useful.

With the introduction of more neonatal screening, whether targeted or not, the role of the HVDT will have to be rethought, its aims sharpened and the testing procedures made less dependent on individual variability/motivation.

Intermediate age surveillance

There is no recommendation to screen children's hearing between 1 year and school entry.[2,13] Increasingly, the reliance will be on appropriate surveillance, eliciting parental concern at each developmental assessment and generating the most effective case-finding strategy. The majority of hearing problems in these age groups are likely to be due to persistent glue ear. I will not deal further with this problem here except to mention that again microprocessor-based implementations of tests such as the McCormick toy test[31,40] may soon be available relatively cheaply for use in primary and community care.

School age screen

The retention of the school age screen is recommended.[2,16] Providing it is monitored correctly, this screen is the last chance in the system for the discovery of congenital and progressive sensorineural hearing impairments. In addition, it may be able to find children with lesser degrees of impairment, e.g. unilateral impairment.

ORGANIZATION OF SERVICES

There are major problems with the organization of hearing screening and allied services in most districts. This is because of the lack of a consistently implemented model for those services and above all the lack of effective coordination. The recommendation of the 'Health for all children'[2] was that 'one person in each district or health board should take responsibility for co-ordinating the programme of hearing screening, including training and refresher courses' (p 66).

I think that this is a good recommendation, but it may no longer be the case that this is practicable in the UK, due to the number of provider trusts that are involved. Rather it seems that the best solution would be if each purchasing district had an 'audiology working party' whose remit was to coordinate hearing services including screening. The chair of such a working party might have a role similar to that advocated above. This is the approach taken in the NDCS quality standards in audiology vol 2.[41]

It is vital that the audiology working party oversees the attainment of the appropriate targets, and collects good quality data on the services provided, possibly with the use of adequate information systems (e.g. PARS). The working party should also pay particular attention to the role of parents (perhaps even on the working party) in child surveillance by encouraging the use of parent-held records containing well-tried questions on hearing and communication at each developmental assessment. The consideration of the parents is essential, particularly in trying to minimize, to some extent, the psychological effects of screening but also to help minimize the impact of diagnosis on the family.[42]

RECOMMENDATIONS: SETTING UP A SCREENING PROGRAMME

1. Before setting up a screening programme there is a need for an audiology working party (AWP) and preferably a named coordinator for hearing screening. Ideally the AWP should have at least one trained professional in audiology (preferably to Master's degree level). The AWP should consider the quality of audiological services, the availability of rehabilitation and the needs of the local community *before* embarking on a new neonatal screening service or radically changing local practice.

2. The aim of the screening programme should be decided by the AWP; for example, to detect all bilaterally permanently hearing impaired children and begin a programme of habilitation for the family and child before the child is at risk of delayed or abnormal cognitive, social and emotional development.

3. More research is needed concerning: (1) what constitutes a material hearing impairment in this context, in terms of severity; (2) what delay can be tolerated before quality of life (for family and child) is materially affected; (3) what interaction there is between severity and delay, for example can mild impairments (say 15–40 dB HL) be left until 4 years with little consequence for later academic achievement and social integration.

4. The AWP in each district should, in the light of present services and the local population, put in place arrangements to carry out a targeted neonatal hearing screen on all at-risk children in line with NDCS quality standards.[16] The preferred method would be either ABR or TEOAE (using the ILO88), but for small numbers where skilled staff are available then ABR may be marginally better. If TEOAE is used there should be an ABR screening or assessment facility to carry out a second screening test. This first step in neonatal screening will provide a considerable public health advantage, at a reasonable cost in recurrent budget terms (£20 000 per year, in 1994, for a district at the median in terms of births per year, i.e. 3337).

5. Due consideration needs to be given to the appropriate audiological training for neonatal screening, and whom to appoint. NICU nurse-managers may require a candidate with neonatal nursing skills. For coverage to be good,

due consideration is needed in terms of adequately topped up high quality training for back-up staffing for holidays, sickness, training and maternity leave.

6. Considerable thought should be given *now* to the introduction in the next few years of universal neonatal screening programmes using TEOAE and conditional ABR. This should be done in the light of the performance of the targeted screen and the HVDT. This step will need very careful planning, so start now. It will have considerable impact in terms of recurrent budget (between £70 000 and £100 000 per year for a typical district) and the screening/surveillance activity in later years. As well as relying on data from the USA, the results of the trial of universal neonatal screening by Dr. Colin Kennedy and colleagues will be an important sign as to future policy.

7. At 6–8 months the HVDT should be continued if there is evidence that it is working. Poor coverage, small yield and low sensitivity suggest that either the strategy should be discontinued or very active retraining is urgently needed. If this leads to massive overreferral this can be just as damaging because it clogs up the system. The major problem will always be monitoring the quality of the work done, due to the nature of the test and the lack of direct scientific audiological line management. Eventually, in this period we should aim to detect those children with mild congenital hearing impairments, but this awaits the development of a hand-held and very quick OAE device.

8. The school sweep audiometry screen has not had the scrutiny that other screening tests in other periods of development have had. Nevertheless, there is general agreement that it should be continued and that it represents good value for money at present. Possibly in the future it may benefit from the use of microprocessor-controlled speech tests that screen for disability rather than impairment.

9. An information/audit strategy is needed for all the screens, especially the above. This may be mandated centrally for each sort of screening activity.[43] However, the requirements outlined in the NDCS quality standards should act as a good starting point.

10. The use of such information technology systems that most easily monitor process measures should not disguise the fact that we need to devise age-standardized outcome measures to properly tune the screening and subsequent intervention strategies. At present they do not exist.

REFERENCES

1 Davis AC. A public health perspective on childhood hearing impairment. In: McCormick B, ed. Paediatric audiology 0–5 years, 2nd ed. London: Whurr Publishers, 1993: pp 1–41
2 Hall DMB. Health for all children: a programme for child health surveillance, 2nd ed. Oxford: Oxford University Press, 1991
3 Joint Committee on Infant Hearing. Position statement 1982. Pediatrics 1982; 70: 496–497
4 Joint Committee on Infant Hearing. Position statement 1990. ASHA 1991; 33 (suppl 5): 3–6

5 National Institutes of Health. Early indentification of hearing impairment in infants and young children. NIH consensus statement vol 11 (No 1, March 1–3). NIH, Bethesda, MD, 1993

6 Fortnum HM, Davis AC. The epidemiology of bacterial meningitis. Arch Dis Child 1993; 68: 763–767

7 Fortnum H, Davis AC. Hearing impairment in children after bacterial meningitis: incidence and resource implications. Br J Audiol 1993; 27: 43–52

8 Fortnum HM. Hearing impairment after bacterial meningitis: a review. Arch Dis Child 1992; 67: 1128–1133

9 Wilson JMG, Jungner G. Principles and practice of screening for disease. Geneva: World Health Organization, 1968

10 Davis AC. Epidemiology of hearing disorders. In: Stephens SDG, ed. Scott-Brown's otolaryngology, 5th ed. vol 2, Adult audiology. Guildford: Butterworth Scientific, 1987: pp 90–126

11 Davis AC, Sancho J. Screening for hearing impairment in children: a review of current practice in the UK with special reference to the screening of babies from special care baby units for severe/profound impairments. In: Gerber SE, Mencher GT, eds. International perspectives on communication disorders. Washington: Gallaudet University Press, 1988: pp 237–275

12 Haggard MP. Research in the development of effective services for hearing-impaired people. London: Nuffield Provincial Hospitals Trust, 1993

13 Haggard MP, Hughes E. Screening children's hearing. London: HMSO, 1991

14 Curnock DA. Identifying hearing impairment in infants and young children. Br Med J 1993; 307: 1225–1226

15 Hall DMB. Health for all children: a programme for child health surveillance. Oxford: Oxford University Press, 1989

16 National Deaf Children's Society. Quality standards in paediatric audiology, vol 1. London: NDCS, 1993

17 Hunter MF, Kimm L, Cafferelli Dees D et al. Feasibility of otoacoustic emission detection followed by ABR as a universal screening test for hearing impairment. Br J Audiol 1994; 28: 47–52

18 White KR, Vohr BR, Behrens TR. Universal newborn hearing screening using transient evoked otoacoustic emissions: results of the Rhode Island hearing assessment project. Semin Hear 1993; 14: 18–29

19 Watkin PM, Baldwin M, Laoide S. Neonatal at risk screening and the identification of deafness. Arch Dis Child 1991; 66: 1130–1135

20 Bennett MJ, Wade HK. Automated newborn screening using the ARC. In: Taylor IE, Markides A, eds. Disorders of auditory function III. London: Academic Press, 1980: pp 59–69

21 Tucker SM, Bhattacharya J. Screening of hearing impairment in the newborn using the auditory response cradle. Arch Dis Child 67: 911–919

22 Mauk GW, Behrens TR. Historical, political, and technological context associated with early identification of hearing loss. Semin Hear 1993; 14: 1–17

23 Davidson J, Hyde ML, Alberti PW. Epidemiologic patterns in childhood hearing loss: a review. Int J Pediatr Otolaryngol 1989; 17: 239–266

24 Davis AC, Wood S. The epidemiology of childhood hearing impairment: factors relevant to the planning of services. Br J Audiol 1992; 26: 77–90

25 Davis AC, Wood S, Webb H et al. Risk factors for childhood hearing disorders. J Am Acad Audiol 1995 (in press)

26 Davis A, Parving A. Towards appropriate epidemiological data on childhood hearing disability: a comparative European study of birth cohorts 1982–88. J Audiol Med 1994; 3: 35–47

27 Summerfield AQ, Marshall D, Davis AC. Demand, cost and utility of cochlear implants. Ann Rhinol Otol Laryngol 1995 (in press)

28 Martin JAM, Bentzen O, Colley SRT et al. Childhood deafness in the European Community. Brussels: Commission of the European Communities, 1979

29 Vanniasegaram I, Tungland OP, Bellman S. A 5-year review of children with deafness in a multiethnic community. J Audiol Med 1993; 2: 9–19

30 Marshall D, Fortnum HM, Davis AC et al. Paediatric Audiology Record System (PARS) manual. IHR internal report series A No 12. Gravesend, Kent: Public Sector Software, 1992

31 McCormick B, ed. Paediatric audiology 0–5 years, 2nd ed. London: Whurr Publishers, 1993

32 Kemp DT. Stimulated acoustic emissions from the human auditory system. J Acoust Soc Am 1978; 64: 1386–1391

33 Thornton ARD, Kimm L, Kennedy CR et al. External and middle ear factors affecting otoacoustic emissions in neonates. Br J Audiol 1993; 27: 319–327

34 Cope Y, Lutman ME. Otoacoustic emissions. In: McCormick B, ed. Paediatric audiology 0–5 years, 2nd ed. London: Whurr Publishers, 1993: pp 250–290

35 Davis AC. The feasibility of using TEOAE for screening at risk neonates. Paper given at 1st International Symposium on Otoacoustic Emissions, Lyons, 1993

36 Mason S. Electric response audiometry. In: McCormick B, ed. Paediatric audiology 0–5 years, 2nd ed. London: Whurr Publishers, 1993: pp 187–249

37 Wharrad H. Neonatal hearing screening tests. In: McCormick B, ed. Paediatric audiology 0–5 years, 1st ed. London: Taylor and Francis, 1988: pp 69–96

38 Simmons FB, Russ FN. Automated newborn hearing screening, the Crib-O-Gram. Arch Otolaryngol 1974; 100: 1–7

39 Scanlon P, Bamford JMB. Early identification of hearing loss: screening and surveillance methods. Arch Dis Child 1990; 65: 470–484

40 Palmer AR, Sheppard S, Marshall DH. Prediction of hearing thresholds in children using an automated toy discrimination test. Br J Audiol 1991; 25: 351–356

41 National Deaf Children's Society. Quality standards in audiology vol II. The audiological management of the child. London: NDCS, 1994

42 Gregory S. The deaf child and his family. London: Allen and Unwin, 1976

43 Haggard MP. Standards in the strategy for developing effective services. In: NDCS quality standards in paediatric audiology. Occasional papers in the field of early identification of hearing impairment in children. London: NDCS, 1995

5. Parental participation in child development centres

P. Appleton

Both the Court Report[1] in 1976, and the Warnock Report[2] in 1978, made strong recommendations concerning the role of parents in services for children with disabilities. Court stressed the need for parents to be treated as participants, not bystanders, in the process of assessment and decision-making. He made the point that it is families that create and sustain the services they require, through electoral and fiscal processes. A whole chapter of the Warnock Report is devoted to the partnership role of parents.

During the 1980s, these specific recommendations for children's services were further reinforced by very significant generic changes in public service philosophy. Patients, or clients, were increasingly seen as customers, who would choose whether to take up services, and should expect to be consulted carefully as to their preferences and wishes.[3] By the mid-1990s this orientation had been enshrined in legislation and, in general terms, had cross-party political support.

The Children Act[4] and the Special Educational Needs (SEN) Code of Practice[5] made parents, and of course the young person him- or herself, central to the planning of care and education. Professionals were seen as having an enabling, not a controlling, role. At the same time as these changes were introduced, a business-oriented philosophy, with stringent financial control, and prevalent use of metaphors such as 'product' and 'package', emerged.[3] Public service staff felt undervalued by Government, and many clinicians found business metaphors distasteful and inappropriate.

It is in this broad social and political context that child development centres (CDCs) have gradually evolved more participatory roles for parents.

Studies of the introduction of changes in CDC practice have been few. Interviews with 50 parents attending an innovative child development service in London showed that a majority felt they had actively selected the type of intervention suited to their child.[6] However, an Oxford regional study of families of 40 children with cerebral palsy found that many parents experienced lack of information and fragmentation of services.[7]

In a Manchester study of 105 families of children with severe physical disabilities, families received an average of 68 professional contacts per year, from an average of ten different disciplines.[8] Frequency of service contact was not associated with degree of unmet need, although it was associated with perceived helpfulness of services. There were a number of areas of unmet need including information about services, and information about the child's condition. Half the sample did not have a 'link person' (to act as a primary contact and to coordinate services), and those that did reported that this was an informal arrangement rather than a systematic part of service policy. Many parents reported that they had to chase progress. A key finding from this study was that high levels of unmet need were associated with life-event strain, child mental handicap, paternal unemployment, and use of passive optimism as a coping strategy by the mother. An overall picture emerges from this study of an inadequate match between service need and service provision. The authors call for greater service accessibility, more provision of information, coordination through a link person, and accurate and individual assessment of family need.

Other studies have also shown that the most vulnerable families are those who are less able to use active coping strategies, and those whose child's condition is severe.[9-11] Some parents experience generalized anxiety, and others experience specific worries concerning the child's capacity to learn independence skills.

The topic of parent–professional cooperation in the care and education of the disabled child may be approached from at least seven different perspectives:

1. Parental responsibility, now enshrined in law (Children Act), empowers parents to take key decisions concerning their child.[4] Professionals are now most appropriately regarded as enablers and advisors, expert in certain aspects of the child's life, providing information, and giving counsel when asked.

2. It is important to remember that what parents of disabled children want from professionals is that they should listen.[12] Listening, and taking careful account of what parents say about their child, and their own circumstances, wishes and beliefs, is the first step in the setting-up of a parent–professional relationship. Much of the 'business' and 'quality' jargon in the 'new' public services hides this simple fact.

3. The development of the parents themselves, as adults as well as parents, is challenged by the tasks of bringing up a child. This may be especially so if the child is disabled. A co-working approach by professionals can safeguard the parents' adult identities, allowing parents to express their own needs, as well as those of their child.[13]

4. Parental care is the primary context for the child's development.[14] Professional care can only be expected, therefore, to have a significant influence on the development of the child, through a process of co-working with parents.

5. There has been concern for some time that poorly coordinated teams of professionals, from different agencies, can act as a set of additional stresses to parents, who are already coping with the demands of caring for the disabled child.[2,3]

6. Involvement of parents in the development, and management, of services, through various mechanisms, is a major theme.[15]

7. Management of change in teams, and interagency networks, is a challenge for services wishing to take parent participation forward.[3,16]

PARENTAL CONTROL OF DECISIONS

Notions of parental responsibility, and participation in decision-making, are central features of the Children Act[4] and the SEN Code of Practice.[5] Parents do not usually wish to be the 'passive recipients of services', even if circumstances make them feel as if they have no power. Most parents wish to participate in making the difficult decisions about surgery, therapies, schooling, and in other key decisions.

Facilitating parents' involvement in decision-making makes good psychological sense. Human beings find uncontrollable situations stressful.[17] If the discovery of a child's disability is compounded by a perceived loss of control over decisions regarding the child, anger and anxiety may result. Some parents report long-term loss of control over decisions affecting medical, educational and social aspects of their child's life. Parent advocacy movements have grown out of hard-won battles between parents and professionals.

Providing information, offering choices, explaining why diagnostic procedures do not always provide clear-cut answers, apologising for errors, and avoidance of jargon, are all important. However, one of the major contributions a professional can make is to communicate that he recognizes the parents' wishes, views, and judgements. The professional may not agree with the parents, but he can respect their autonomy and responsibility.

The word 'empowerment' is frequently used to describe, amongst other things, the recognition of parental autonomy.[18] An unfortunate connotation of the word is the implication that professionals are able to grant, or give, initiative to parents. In fact, in the eyes of the law, parents are wholly responsible for their child's care, and for decisions pertaining to that care.[4] Psychologically, the parents and child may benefit from the perception that they are supported in their autonomous roles, and in turn may seek the views of professionals more readily, in order to make more informed decisions. It is also to be hoped that parents will perceive fewer barriers to their plans, and begin to regard professionals as there to enable and assist. Some parents may have experienced their own schooling as not meeting their needs, others may still be learning to cope with information about their child's condition, or may have experienced a long sequence of 'uncontrollable events'. Yet others may have experienced chronic stress caring for a young person with severe physical or intellectual impairments. In each of these cases the setting-up of a parent–professional relationship will require time and patient listening.[19] A key aim of that relationship is that the parents will experience more readily their own democratic freedom.

THE PARENT–PROFESSIONAL RELATIONSHIP

Active and reflective listening by the professional can establish a parent–professional relationship that enables free interchange of views, provision of appropriate help, lowered parental anxiety, and greater appreciation by the parent of his/her own capacities and skills.[12,19]

The process of active listening is not always easy to establish in busy clinics, but may prevent unnecessary duplication of effort, reduce inappropriate dependency on services, reduce parental anxiety, and increase precision of diagnosis and assessment. A frequent complaint by parents is that they were not heard.

It is during the assessment and diagnostic phase that active listening can be most helpful.[20] During this phase of heightened parental sensitivity, parents are at greatest need of sympathetic and accurate listening. Open questions, and elicitation of expectations, fears and hopes, are useful. A non-judgemental approach is essential. History-taking should be broad-based, allowing parental priorities, and attitudes, to be expressed and acknowledged.

When developmental tests are administered with the child, it is useful to share with the parents those observations which tally with their own, thus reinforcing parental confidence. It is important to acknowledge that situational factors affect a child's performance on tests. A 'joint approach' to discovering the child's strengths and difficulties will be appreciated, and may produce more precise results.

Feedback of assessment results also requires a listening stance, checking whether parents have understood, and checking whether they agree. The tendency to formality of a 'case review' is not conducive to this type of communication. Parents need the opportunity to check out perceptions in a psychologically safe setting such as their own home, or in a very small meeting. They then need an opportunity to digest assessment findings, before planning interventions.

Parent–professional relationships established within this framework are less likely to be characterized by inappropriate hostility. Clearly some parents will feel angry about their child's disability and may feel safe to express that. Anger is less likely to be directed at the professional, or the decision-making process, if the parents have felt consulted, and feel involved in decisions.

Relationships can, of course, be too close. Establishing an optimal distance is important, not being so close as to strangle objectivity, and not so far as to freeze genuine and warm emotional support.[21]

While it is true that a parent may go through stages when a particular professional is an extremely important source of information and support, nevertheless for most of the child's development the most important parental relationships are those of family and friends. It is always helpful for the professional to decentre from the parent–professional relationship and to consider how to enable informal support to provide for needs.

ADULT DEVELOPMENT

The development of the parents themselves, as adults as well as parents, is challenged by the tasks of caring for children.[14] This may be especially so if a child is disabled. A co-working approach by professionals can safeguard the parents' adult identities, allowing parents to express their own needs, as well as those of their children.

Studies of services which utilize parents as therapists have shown that such interventions can be counterproductive if the parent's own needs are overlooked.[22] Some parents may experience developmental programmes, which they have to administer, as additional stresses. Other parents may take on supervised developmental programmes with alacrity, making their own needs of secondary importance. This is not always to the benefit of the child, or family. The parent may invest high hopes, and especial importance, in successful outcomes. The child may experience undue pressure, and may resist, thus setting up negative cycles. In turn the parent may lose self-esteem, having invested her concept of herself, as an adult, in successfully promoting the child's development.

The parent's sense of herself as a 'good parent' may have been undermined by the child's disability status. Engaging in developmental programmes may be compensatory for the parent. Using a co-working approach, professionals can try to reach a balanced care and education plan, utilizing parenting strengths, but also recognizing adult needs.

Important practical steps can be taken to ensure, during the assessment phase, that parents can see a professional on their own, without the demanding presence of the child. In these circumstances parents need to feel confident that the child is being well cared for, and that they can relax.

A parent may have mixed feelings about her working arrangements, feeling on the one hand that work brings money in and gives her adult space and identity, yet on the other hand takes her away from her child. Such dilemmas are made more complex when the child has a disability. Active and reflective listening by a professional can be helpful, especially when the parents may be receiving strong and conflicting advice from family and friends. It is not useful to partition out adult development issues as solely the province of one professional discipline. Disciplines working more with the children's needs can feel frustrated with parents, and can undermine parents by subtle communication of that frustration. Adult development is everybody's business because, at least in the early years, the parents are usually the child's main, consistent, long-term resource.

Group-work for parents of disabled children may be helpful, but evaluations suggest caution.[11] The purposes must be well-defined. Will the group concentrate on parenting, or on adult emotional and life-skills issues? If concentrating on adult issues, will the group have a curriculum of skill-based work (e.g. assertiveness, problem-solving, elicitation of appropriate support), or will it be more exploratory? Evaluation of attendance, acceptability, and skill outcome is essential.

The first three sections of this paper have concentrated almost entirely on adult or parental issues. Children have hardly been mentioned. The purpose of this has been to draw attention to the level of detail required in considering parental participation in CDCs. Whereas CDCs have comprehensive and thorough methods for investigating the child's disability, less detailed attention has been paid to the process of establishing relationships with the child's main developmental resource, the parents. Participation by parents in the care and education of their children, and in the planning of services, is only possible in the context of relationships characterized by mutual respect, reciprocal sharing of information and skills and feelings, shared decision-making, and recognition of individuality.[23]

These principles are more important than techniques such as parent-held records, information packs, or parental attendance at case reviews. Such techniques, if implemented independently of an overall policy review of parental participation, may only have a 'token' function.

SUPPORTING PARENTAL CARE

One of the most useful changes in perspective to have emerged over the last few years is that of taking what is known about parenting, and applying that knowledge to the understanding of parental care of disabled children.[11] Until recently, professionals, and researchers, had tended to aim to specify what was abnormal, or pathological, about parents of disabled children. The new perspective does not deny that parenting a child with significant impairments can be highly stressful. Instead it aims to specify what the significant stresses are, what naturalistic coping adaptations parents make, and what informal sources of support are drawn on.[10,24] Such a knowledge base can then clear the way to specify how services can be designed to support and extend existing parental coping strategies. Research using this perspective is still at an early stage, but there is wide agreement that the perspective is clinically useful, and acceptable to parents.

Personal coping resources and skills include the parents' physical and psychological health, beliefs and attitudes, capacity and skills in parenting the child, preferred coping strategies in stressful conditions, and personality. Social resources include available social support, spouse support, economic and employment circumstances, and formal support from public service or voluntary agencies.[10]

For CDCs three themes from recent research are striking. First, it is important, where possible, to involve both parents. Each may have different needs,[13] and each will have a different relationship to the child.[8] For two-parent families the most important source of support to the main carer is usually the spouse.[10] Services can attempt to reinforce the support by working with both parents. For one-parent families the parent may identify someone who is close, and may wish to be included in professional consultations. Secondly, central to the child's development is the nature of his relationships with his parents.[14] It is these relationships which motivate, teach, protect, and give joy. At each stage of the young person's development, different tasks are required from parents. Professionals need to assess how they can substantively support the primary resources the child has. In the assessment phase parents can make systematic observations of the child's behaviour and development, in partnership with professionals.[20] In the therapeutic phase, for preschool children there may be benefit to work on mutual communication of intention and understanding.[11] For adolescents, parents may wish to work on helping the young person appropriately and gradually to detach, and become independently capable.

In a prospective study of interventions for 190 developmentally disabled infants in the USA, data underscored the need for early intervention services to focus on the parent–child relationship.[11] At the time of entry into the programme (mean age at entry 10.6 months) infants showed delayed interactive behaviours. In comparison with parents of age-matched infants without disabilities, fathers experienced more stress in feelings of attachment to infants, and mothers experienced more difficulty in reading the children's signals, and facilitating learning. Mother–child interactions remained problematic after 12 months of intervention. Qualities of relationships do not improve automatically, and disrupted parent–child interactions are a risk factor for behavioural problems. There is a large body of mainstream work in the developmental psychology of early childhood which has only recently been applied to the study of developmental delay. Intervention studies focusing on parent–child interaction are urgently needed.[11] Thirdly, most studies have shown that parents are hungry for information about the child's condition.[13] Similar issues apply as to the provision of information about services

CARE COORDINATION

If parents are to exercise responsibility in the planning, and giving, of care and education for their child, then some type of coordination or management of interdisciplinary professional services is necessary.[3,8,25] The family's coordinator of care will need the authority and skills to liaise effectively with all disciplines and agencies, and to draw up care and education plans. The Manchester study drew attention to the patchiness of such initiatives.[8] Named care coordinators should have certain key functions:

1. The establishment of relationships of partnership with parents based on principles outlined earlier in this paper.
2. To act as a focal point of multiprofessional service contact for the family, recognized by both family and service providers.
3. To actively help the parents develop their roles in understanding, meeting, and representing the child's individual needs.

4. To actively help parents to represent their own unique wishes, preferences, and needs.
5. To provide continuity, as well as coordination, of multiprofessional care.

Multiprofessional services refers not only to the particular CDC that the child attends, but also to all relevant services. Team-assigned care coordinators, or key workers, may confine their roles largely to intrateam coordination, when for many families the greatest need for coordination may be between services or teams. This is particularly the case for coordination between schools and CDCs.[26] The focus of attention of the coordinator must be through the eyes of the family, not the eyes of the team.

The role cannot be a reactive one. The points about the development of a relationship have been made. A review system, with multiprofessional clinical audit, based on client pathways, may be helpful. The provision of information is critical. Each profession may assume that another discipline has provided information. The parents may not know what information they need. Such gaps require coordination of function.[3]

The care coordinator is in a strong position to adjust the provision of care to parents' literacy and intellectual levels. Parents with a history of educational disadvantage may feel uneasy with all written communications, and may miss appointments, or feel unable to disclose views and opinions. Misunderstandings can easily arise. While a proportion of parents will feel competent to use public libraries and voluntary organizations to seek information, others will feel both isolated by lack of information, and low in confidence to ask questions. Twelve per cent of young adults report literacy problems.[27] In general, prevalence of literacy problems will be higher amongst parents of children with intellectual impairments, given what is known of intergenerational continuities in intellectual and educational attainment.[28] The area of literacy, and parental participation, is worthy of systematic research.

In a study of written information provided by 11 CDCs in the West Midlands, many leaflets were considered difficult for parents to understand.[29] The authors recommend the use of Flesch formulae, and the involvement of parents in the writing of leaflets. The importance of sensitivity to cultural and ethnic issues, and the provision of information in the first language of parents, were emphasized.

Transitions important for the family may require special coordinative help. Guidance documents mark out early preparation for transition to adult services, and this is a welcome move.[5] But individual families may give weight to other transitions, such as entry into playgroup, entry into school, start or loss of parental employment, start or loss of adult relationships, developmental transitions, or a move to another part of the country. There is a considerable literature suggesting that help-giving is more effective if it is based on a careful assessment of precisely what the parents want, and their personal, individual styles of coping.[19]

Since Warnock's recommendation of a named person for each child with special needs, there has been general recognition of the need for families to have a single point of contact.[2] Unfortunately, the various functions which such a role may involve — coordination, counselling, advocacy, care management — leave room for vagueness and lack of precise local policy development. The new SEN Code of Practice may not help in this regard.[5] It is recommended that both a Local Education Authority (LEA) named person, and a non-LEA named person be involved in educational statementing. The central, client-centred requirement for overall coordination, and active listening, may not be met by these recommendations.

PARENTAL PARTICIPATION IN SERVICE PLANNING

Part of the landscape of political change in the 1980s and 1990s has been not only the participation of parents in individual care planning, but also in general service planning. User participation in social service settings, parents as governors in schools, and parents as part of service planning groups in the National Health Service and local government, is now customary.[15] It is part of the political drive to make public services appear more accountable and service-oriented. As, during the 1990s, difficult questions of resource priority become progressively more explicit, there will be an increased perceived need for public participation in service planning and policy-making. Parents will be consulted by commissioners of health and social care for children, and new forms of public representation to advise commissioners will be established.

Sometimes independently of professional input, parents of disabled children make parent-to-parent links which provide important support.[10] Professionals can facilitate this type of initiative, and other forms of self-help, which may form into advocacy and pressure groups. Parents may wish to become involved in time-limited projects such as the writing of a leaflet, the design stage of research, or quality development work. Ideally, parents are much needed on policy development groups, and CDC management groups. Our experience has been that parents, irrespective of the age of the child or young person, find it very difficult to sustain attendance at regular meetings. Our services have benefited greatly from short-term involvement of parents on projects, or on groups, but it is unreasonable to expect parents to put a high personal priority on extended involvement. Some parents feel they see enough of professionals, without voluntarily increasing the contact. Other parents feel that they cannot truly represent the views of other parents.

A personal view is that, if the principles of individual parent–professional relationships outlined above are developed in an organization, then there is a process of continuous feedback from parents. Service deficits are highlighted, and service developments, initiated jointly by parents and professionals, can develop using available resources, which can, when possible, include parents.

MAKING IT HAPPEN

CDCs wishing to take forward participation with parents may initially be overwhelmed by the number of changes that may need to be made. Preconditions for implementation include:

1. Appropriate staff development and training.
2. Agreement by staff and managers on service policy changes.
3. Clarity of staff management arrangements for implementation of policy.
4. Clarity of links with other agencies, particularly schools, to ensure coordination of parental participation.
5. A mechanism for routine audit of the quality of parental participation, from the point of view of parents.
6. A plan for introducing systematic care coordination.

While it may seem overwhelming, the implementation of a parent participation strategy is a means of addressing, at the same time, a number of other key issues in CDCs. To take two examples: quality assurance initiatives clearly must involve parents,[30] and improvement of interdisciplinary working may be easier when focused on an undeniably important task such as the achievement of effective parental participation.[3]

The time-scale for change must be realistic. Training, new assessment and treatment mechanisms, change in communication and coordination mechanisms, and management changes, all take time. A 3-year programme of incremental steps is reasonable, and must of course be flexible in the light of the continuous flux experienced in modern public service agencies. Leadership is essential, with an emphasis on the drawing together, by a common aim, of otherwise disparate disciplines.

With a clear purpose, time brings opportunities which can all be drawn into the long-term goal. Each new member of staff appointed can be made aware, through job description and interview discussion, of the high profile of parental participation. Students on placement can be encouraged to do appropriate evaluations. Finally, commissioners of health and social care for children are in a strong position to induce organizational change through service specifications.

KEY POINTS FOR CLINICAL PRACTICE

- Parental responsibility is a central feature of the Children Act. Enabling parents to make informed decisions concerning their child's care and education is a key role of CDCs.
- Although the establishment of healthy parent–professional relationships is time-consuming, requiring skilled listening and sensitive information-giving, there should be considerable clinical benefits to the child and family, and probably a saving of resources in the long-term.
- Parent–professional co-working should begin during the early stages of assessment and diagnosis.

- Understanding parents own needs, and enabling them to meet those needs, is an important function of CDCs.
- Appropriate steps should be taken to involve both parents, or others nominated by the main carer, in respect of decisions, and the implementation of assessment and care/education plans.
- Fragmentation of service provision is an avoidable additional stress to families. CDCs are in a strong position to provide named coordinators of care/education for individual children, and their families.
- Parents should be offered the opportunity of involvement in policy and service development initiatives. Certain initiatives, such as the writing of CDC leaflets, or design and piloting of consumer satisfaction instruments, are, by definition, unlikely to be satisfactory if parents are not directly involved in determining content and methods.
- The management of the design and implementation of policies of parental participitation in CDCs requires the same degree of clarity, explicitness and forward-planning as does the individual child's diagnosis, assessment and care/education planning.

ACKNOWLEDGEMENTS

I wish to acknowledge many discussions with parents, and with my colleagues Vicki Böll, Dr Adele Kelly, Kate Meredith, Dr Philip Minchom, Peter Reid and Brian Stickels.

REFERENCES

1 Department of Health. Fit for the future. Report of the Committee on Child Health Services. London: HMSO, 1976
2 Department of Education and Science. Report of the Committee of Enquiry into the education of handicapped children and young people. London: HMSO, 1978
3 Øvretveit J. Coordinating community care: multidisciplinary teams and care management. Buckingham: Open University Press, 1993
4 Department of Health. The Children Act 1989 guidance and regulations. Children with disabilities. London: HMSO, 1991: vol 6
5 Department for Education. Code of Practice on the identification and assessment of special educational needs. London: Central Office of Information, 1994
6 Dale NJ. Parental involvement in the KIDS Family Centre: who does it work for? Child Care Health Dev 1992; 18: 301–319
7 Haylock CL, Johnson MA, Harpin VA. Parents' views of community care for children with motor disabilities. Child Care Health Dev 1993; 19: 209–220
8 Sloper P, Turner S. Service needs of families of children with severe physical disability. Child Care Health Dev 1992; 18: 259–282
9 Frey KS, Greenberg MT, Fewell RR. Stress and coping among parents of handicapped children: a multidimensional approach. Am J Ment Retard 1989; 94: 240–249
10 Beresford BA. Resources and strategies: how parents cope with the care of a disabled child. J Child Psychol Psychiatry 1994; 35: 171–209
11 Shonkoff JP, Hauser-Cram P, Krauss MW, Upshur CC. Development of infants with disabilities and their families: implications for theory and service delivery. Monogr Soc Res Child Dev 1992; 57 (No. 6, Serial No. 230)
12 Cunningham C, Davis H. Working with parents: frameworks for collaboration. Milton Keynes: Open University Press, 1985

13 Bailey DB, Blasco PM, Simeonsson RJ. Needs expressed by mothers and fathers of young children with disabilities. Am J Ment Retard 1992; 97: 1–10
14 Bronfenbrenner U. The ecology of human development: experiments by nature and design. London: Harvard University Press, 1979
15 Lupton C, Hall B. Beyond the rhetoric: from policy to practice in user-involvement. Res Policy Planning 1993; 10: 6–11
16 Appleton PL. Working together for young children: parent partnership and multidisciplinary teams. Paper given at Third Annual Conference of the Clwyd Association for the Development of Young Children, 1987
17 Brewin, C. Cognitive foundations of clinical psychology. London: Lawrence Erlbaum, 1988
18 Appleton PL, Minchom PE. Models of parent partnership and child development centres. Child Care Health Dev 1991; 17: 27–38
19 Dunst C, Trivette C, Deal A. Enabling and empowering families: principles and guidelines for practice. Cambridge, MA: Brookline Books, 1988
20 Parker SJ, Zuckerman BS. Therapeutic aspects of the assessment process. In: Meisels SJ, Shonkoff JP, eds. Handbook of early childhood intervention. Cambridge: Cambridge University Press, 1990
21 Foley GM, Hochman JD, Miller S. Parent–professional relationships: finding on optimal distance. Zero to Three 1994; 14: 19–22
22 McConachie HR. Home-based teaching: what are we asking of parents? Child Care Health Dev 1991; 17: 123–136
23 Mittler P, Mittler H. Partnership with parents: an overview. In: Mittler P, McConachie H, eds. Parents, professionals and mentally handicapped people: approaches to partnership. London: Croom Helm, 1984: p 8–43
24 McConachie H. Implications of a model of stress and coping for services to families of young disabled children. Child Care Health Dev 1994; 20: 37–46
25 Moxley DP. The practice of case management. London: Sage, 1989
26 Eiser C, Town C. Teachers' concerns about chronically sick children: implications for paediatricians. Dev Med Child Neurol 1987; 29: 56–63
27 Ferri E, ed. Life at 33: the fifth follow-up of the National Child Development Study. London: National Childrens Bureau, 1993
28 Rutter M, Madge N. Cycles of disadvantage. London: Heinemann, 1976
29 Reed J, Conneely J, Gorham P, Coxhead S. Assessing the written information given to families prior to their attendance at a child development centre. Child Care Health Dev 1993; 19: 317–325
30 Krahn GL, Eisert D, Fifield B. Obtaining parental perceptions of the quality of services for children with special health needs. J Pediatr Psychol 1990; 6: 761–774

6. Preschool vision screening

G.J. Laing

In 1989 the Joint Working Party on Child Health Surveillance published its report 'Health for all children'.[1] After reviewing the surveillance programme for visual impairment, the working party decided that there was no conclusive evidence to support an extensive screening programme and recommended that 'screening for visual defects in preschool children should be confined to history and observation'; 2 years later the second edition restated this view.[2] The report recommended that neonatal examination should include a careful inspection of the eyes and that parents should be asked about a family history of visual disorders and about their child's visual behaviour at initial and subsequent contacts. It commented that the coverage of screening remains low and the false positive rate of referrals unacceptably high. In addition, the benefits of early diagnosis and treatment in terms of significant clinical improvement remain unclear.

Despite these problems many districts continue to screen children for visual defects in the preschool period. There is considerable variation in the screening methods and personnel.[3,4]

Screening programmes should detect disorders at an early stage when prevention or effective treatment can be achieved. They are generally recommended for conditions that are considered to be important and serious both to professionals and to the community. Severe visual defects are rare and usually present with abnormal visual behaviour. The preschool vision screening programme aims to identify children with the commoner but less serious visual disorders of squint, amblyopia and refractive error.

THE DEVELOPMENT OF VISUAL FUNCTION

Significant changes in visual function and acuity take place during the first 6 months of life.[5] Normal development of the retina and occipital cortex depends on adequate stimulation and correct alignment of the eyes during early infancy. If the developing visual system is deprived of an adequate stimulus or receives conflicting information due to strabismus, anisometropia or amblyopia, the brain may suppress information and normal maturation does not occur. The first 2 years of life appear to be a critical period for the development of the visual pathway and effective binocular vision, although there is some residual plasticity until about 6 years of age. After this time the impairment of visual acuity is likely to become irremediable.

The visual acuity of the newborn has been estimated as 6/240, developing to 6/18–6/6 by 6 months of age.[5] There are marked individual differences, with some 2-month-old infants having acuities as high as 6/24. Estimates obtained from visual evoked responses are higher than those obtained from behavioural methods[6] and it is not yet possible to state at precisely what age adult acuity is reached. Children may demonstrate 6/6 acuity with single letter targets but have difficulty with linear charts and up to 40% of 3–4½-year-olds may not have reached adult acuity for a linear display.[7] Statistical modelling has been used to establish age-related standards for visual acuity using the Sonksen Silver Acuity System.[8] From these, it has been estimated that 90% of 3–4-year-olds will achieve an acuity of 3/4.5. An acuity of 3/3 was not reached by 90% of children until the age of 5.7 years. Infants are normally hypermetropic but show a preferential response for objects at close range. A high degree of hypermetropia has been shown to be associated with the development of a convergent squint and with amblyopia.[9,10]

SEVERE VISUAL IMPAIRMENT

The prevalence of severe visual impairment in early childhood is estimated as 3–4 per 10 000 births.[11] Children with disabilities are at greater risk of visual disorders which may not be diagnosed, so that case ascertainment of severe visual disorder may be incomplete in this group. Cataract, glaucoma and retinoblastoma are surgically treatable and other conditions have genetic implications. Many infants with serious visual problems have obvious ocular abnormalities or abnormal eye movements which are noticed by parents and health professionals in the first few weeks of life.[12] Other children are in high-risk groups and are likely to be identified following referral for specialist visual assessment. The majority of children with severe visual impairment have been identified prior to, and independently of, the universal screening programme.[13]

Refractive errors

Visual acuity is a measure of the ability to separate adjacent visual stimuli and is dependent on both the cerebral cortex and the eyes. A refractive error leads to an unclear image being formed on the retina and retinoscopy is required for direct measurement of that error. The degree of refractive error can be assessed by the measurement of visual acuity and the Snellen letter chart is the criterion against which all other acuity charts are standardized.

Measurements of refraction in a childhood population form an approximately normal distribution with no clear dividing line between normal and abnormal. The acuity result obtained will vary according to the use of actual or behavioural methods. In young children it is difficult to differentiate between blurred vision due to amblyopia and that due to refractive error. It is therefore difficult to ascertain the prevalence of refractive errors in preschool children. Hypermetropia, anisometropia (a difference in refraction between the two eyes) and astigmatism probably occur in 10–15% of infants.[14] Acquired myopia rarely presents before the age of 6 years and the prevalence then increases throughout the school years.[11]

There is no test currently available for screening visual acuity in very young children. The Stycar vision tests were developed for visual assessment in young and handicapped children and are not recommended for screening.[13] Several methods, including 1 mm 'hundreds and thousands', are used to assess visual behaviour. When tested with each eye individually, infants with impairment may object strongly to occlusion of their non-affected eye. Behaviour tests are often used in an imprecise fashion without clear pass–fail criteria and children with a moderate loss of near visual acuity will easily pick up a 1 mm sweet.[7,13] By about 3 years of age it becomes possible to screen children's visual acuity with modified versions of adult testing charts. Snellen charts were designed with a standard spacing between each letter, but the original letter matching charts for children do not conform to this standard. Newer systems such as the Sonksen–Silver Acuity System, Egan Calver and the Cambridge crowded cards do present correctly spaced letters.

Visual acuity should be measured for each eye separately and acceptance of occlusion steadily increases with age; 90% of 3-year-olds can be tested with both eyes together and 80% will tolerate occlusion.[7,15] Occluders in use include a Dermacel patch, glasses with a blackened lens, a 'pirate patch' or a crumpled tissue in mother's hand.

Even small errors of refraction are associated with both amblyopia and squints. However, the effectiveness of treatment of refractive errors in preschool children when there is no association with squint or amblyopia is unknown and the point at which treatment becomes beneficial is uncertain. Minor refractive errors in older children appear to have little impact on education, performance or behaviour and the benefits of prescribing spectacles for this group of children, who often choose not to wear them, are unclear.[16,17]

Squint (strabismus)

Squints (strabismus) occur when the visual axis of one eye is not directed at the same point of visual fixation as the other. They are due to a defect in the binocular fixation reflexes that normally enable the two eyes to work together to perceive a single stereoscopic picture. Children rapidly overcome the resulting double vision by suppressing the central vision of the deviating eye and this leads to the development of amblyopia.

The prevalence at 7 years of age is estimated as 3.5%.[11] Children are at increased risk if they have other disabilities, were of low birthweight or have a family history of squint: 18% of premature babies may develop a squint in later childhood.[3]

Squints are comparatively uncommon during early infancy but can develop between 3 and 6 months of age.[18] There is usually a large constant deviation which is not associated with an appreciable refractive error. Most childhood squints are convergent with an onset between 18 months and 3 years of age and many are associated with a refractive error, commonly hypermetropia.[19] A full range of ocular movements is maintained and the angle of squint is the same in all positions of gaze. Squints typically appear initially on near fixation, particularly when the child is tired and the deviation ranges from being hardly detectable to cosmetically obvious. It may be intermittent or constant. There is considerable variation in the age of presentation of squint in different studies.[3,20] Both convergent and divergent squints may also be the presenting sign of serious ocular or systemic disease.

Squints can sometimes be detected by careful observation and inspection of corneal reflections. In other cases a cover and prism test will be necessary for diagnosis. These tests are more difficult to perform to a high standard and a cover test will not detect microstrabismus. Paralytic squints are identified by testing ocular movements in all positions of gaze. A true squint does not resolve spontaneously, but pseudosquints due to prominent epicanthic folds may be a source of confusion and false positive diagnosis.

Ineffective or late treatment of a squint may be associated with social and educational problems which persist into adulthood.[3] When clumsy children and those with non-specific learning difficulties are excluded, 7-year-olds with a squint tend to have more reading problems and difficulty in copying designs than those without a squint.[11]

There is controversy about the natural history of squints but the aim of treatment is to promote or restore binocular function and prevent the development or reduce the severity of amblyopia. If this cannot be achieved, a cosmetically satisfactory appearance should be attained. Management includes the treatment of amblyopia with occlusion, the correction of any refractive error and surgical correction of the deviation where necessary.

Amblyopia

Amblyopia is 'a reduction in visual acuity for which no organic cause can be detected by physical examination of the eye', or 'defective visual acuity which persists after correction of the refractive error and removal of any pathological obstacle to vision'. Amblyopia is associated with the presence, in the developing visual system, of strabismus, refractive errors (most commonly hypermetropia and anisometropia) and form or stimulus deprivation due to cataract or corneal scarring. It causes an irreversible loss of functional vision (unilateral or bilateral) which cannot be corrected with spectacles.

It is a common condition in childhood and estimates of prevalence range from 1% to 5%.[3,21] There is no consistent definition of the level of vision that constitutes amblyopia and the criterion of no better than 6/9 in the 'bad' eye does not fully reflect the degree of amblyopia. A more than one line difference on a Snellen chart has been suggested as an alternative, provided that the better eye is no worse than 6/9. The average age of onset is difficult to ascertain but it has been assumed generally that refractive errors precede and cause amblyopia.[22] Infants who are markedly hypermetropic are 20 times more likely to develop both strabismus and persisting amblyopia.[5]

Screening children to prevent the development of amblyopia relies on early detection of the associated squint or refractive error. Despite the preschool vision screening programme, most children with amblyopia are not identified until after school entry and there has been no significant improvement in the age at which amblyopia is detected, in the prevalence or severity of the condition.[10,20,23] Amblyopia associated with a squint is more likely to be detected early and failure to identify the straight-eyed amblyope may be partially explained by use of a single letter test. Over 20 years ago it was recognized that the single optotype Sheridan Gardiner test may fail to identify children with amblyopia[24] but this test remains in use in many centres. When the 'crowding phenomenon' occurs, single letter acuity may be normal or near normal, but affected children cannot distinguish a row of adjacent letters and it is only when linear acuity is tested that amblyopia becomes apparent. Crowded card systems were developed to overcome this problem.

Amblyopia is almost always unilateral. Screening for a unilateral loss may not be justifiable although it does result in a loss of true binocular vision and the ability to perceive depth accurately. This may limit an individual's ability to drive, to reach their full potential in sporting activities and their eligibility for certain occupations. Decreased depth perception also puts the other eye at increased risk of injury and results in 25 people becoming blind each year in the UK.[25] There may also be other effects and analysis of data collected by the Child Health and Education Study found an association between marked amblyopia and lower intelligence and sports scores which may or may not be causal.[17]

The principle of treatment is to promote the use of the amblyopic eye by compromising the vision of the better eye. This usually requires occlusion together with correction of any refractive error. Amblyopia can develop in the initially non-amblyopic eye and part-time occlusion is preferred to full-time.[18] The value of occlusion has not been tested scientifically and reported success rates vary from 77% to 100%. Success is thought to relate to the age of onset and presentation, the length of stimulus deprivation and the presence of abnormal hypermetropia as an infant.[9,10,18] Compliance with occlusion and spectacle wearing is often a problem, especially when the amblyopia is dense, but toleration is greater when intervention is commenced in infancy. The results of treatment are often modest with an improvement of one or two lines on the Snellen chart. Amblyopia may recur soon after the cessation of treatment and require further periods of occlusion. Recurrence occasionally occurs at 12–13 years of age.

It has been proposed that some cases of amblyopia could be prevented by identifying and treating children with severe hypermetropia in infancy, but there remains uncertainty as to the effect of early correction on the future development of amblyopia.[9,10,26]

EVALUATION OF VISION SCREENING PROGRAMMES

Evaluation of a screening programme should consider the potential costs, benefits and outcome for individuals, for the health service and for the population as a whole. Evaluation of vision screening is complicated by uncertainty about the natural history of visual development and defects as well as the benefits of early intervention. In addition, doubts have been raised about problems which may be inherent in the tests themselves. Several studies have been designed to ascertain the characteristics of the screening tests and the overall performance of the programme. This section reviews a selection of published studies.

Ingram attempted to determine the extent to which vision screening would satisfy the Wilson and Junger screening criteria.[10] Children in Northamptonshire were seen at 3½ years by an orthoptist (cover and visual acuity tests) and then independently by an ophthalmologist (refraction). The coverage rate was 70%. Children were followed up to 5 or 11 years of age, depending on their age at the start of the study. One-quarter of children with abnormal vision had presented prior to screening and 41% were identified by testing. One-third presented at a later stage and of these nearly half had apparently normal vision when screened. The rest either did not attend or were not known to be living in the district at the time. The study concludes that further assessment of screening should be undertaken and that although testing at 3½ years does detect a considerable proportion of children with visual defects it must be followed by additional case finding.

Community-based orthoptists in Cornwall are using a combination of tests including Snellen or Sheridan Gardiner charts and prisms to examine children at around 4 years of age.[27] A sensitivity (proportion of true positives correctly identified) of 90% was estimated from identifying 'missed cases' when they started school. The specificity (proportion of true negatives correctly identified) was obtained from comparing the screening results with the hospital diagnosis and was estimated at 99%. The positive predictive value (proportion of screen positives who are true positives) was 94% and the negative predictive value was 99%. These results are encouraging but the report does not mention the coverage of screening and only includes those children who attended for preschool and school appointments.

Contrasting results were obtained by an audit of preschool vision screening by clinical medical officers (CMOs).[28] Sixty-three per cent of the target population had been screened at 3½ years with a Stycar five letter test and the

Stycar seven letter test was used as a reference test at school entry. The sensitivity of the preschool screen was estimated as 77%, the specificity as 96% and the positive predictive value as 50%. This study re-emphasizes that unsatisfactory results are obtained with single letter tests and notes that accurate record keeping was also a problem. An unknown proportion of the 'false negatives' may have developed amblyopia and refractive errors between initial screening and school entry.

An earlier South London study estimated the characteristics of several tests used in vision screening using the Snellen chart as the reference test.[13] Out of the five methods tested only the Stycar seven letter test gave satisfactory results although the severity of amblyopia was underestimated. The sensitivity for detection of moderate and severe defects was 98–100%. The specificity was 64%.

A study in Avon examined the referral and detection rates of screening and compared these when orthoptists or CMOs were used as the primary screeners.[29] Both groups used the cover test and Sheridan Gardiner cards but the orthoptists also used prism testing and a test of three-dimensional visual perception. The amblyopia detection rate from orthoptists was 11/1000, which was significantly higher than that of 5/1000 from CMOs. The squint detection rate was 11/1000 compared with 3/1000. The false positive referral rate was also significantly higher in the cohort screened by CMOs. One disadvantage of the orthoptist screening programme was a coverage rate of 73% compared with 85% for a 3½-year check which included vision screening by a CMO. The authors note the additional costs of providing an orthoptic screening programme although other authors comment that the introduction of a secondary level community orthoptic service may reduce the number of costly outpatient visits and become cost effective.[30] It may also be associated with a reduction in the number of false positive referrals and a decrease in waiting times.

A screening test must be safe and acceptable to parents, children and staff as well as being relatively quick and easy to perform. In most areas vision testing takes place as part of the surveillance programme. Assessment of acuity at the 3 + year check takes between 4 and 12 minutes to administer.[7,10] The use of orthoptists as primary screeners often requires an additional visit by parents and includes additional tests which take about 10 minutes when the child is cooperative.[27]

One of the criticisms of the screening programme is that there has been no apparent decrease in the prevalence or severity of subsequent vision problems.[10] A Canadian study aimed to determine whether a kindergarten screening programme affected the prevalence of vision problems 6–12 months later, using a non-screened cohort as a control group.[31] The results were encouraging. Screening with the Illiterate E test was associated with half as many vision problems overall, and a 79% reduction in moderate to severe vision problems. The random selection of children into a screened or non-screened control group may present ethical problems in areas where screening is well established.

Screening might also result in a peak in the number of children identified with target conditions at the age of screening. A survey in Kettering reviewed all cases referred to hospital and school clinics over a 1-year period.[20] There were two peaks in the referral age for squint, at 3–4 and at 5–6 years. Half of the squints presented after 5 years of age and were often not cosmetically noticeable. There was no preschool peak for amblyopia and two-thirds of cases presented after the age of 5 years. A similar study also describes the age of presentation of new cases of amblyopia in an area where children are screened at 3½ years of age with the single letter Sheridan Gardiner test.[23] Only 15% of amblyopic children without a squint presented before 5 years of age. In both studies children with associated squints were identified earlier.

A London-based audit aimed to assess whether the screening programme was functioning efficiently and considered the appropriateness of referrals.[32] Data were collected about children who were referred to ophthalmology clinics following screening. Children were examined for squints with corneal reflections and cover test and visual acuity was estimated at that time with the Stycar five letter test. Out of 184 referrals, 55% were considered to be justifiable but only 20% had a clear visual defect. Problems were also identified in the non-attendance rate at the clinic following referral (20%) and delays between screening and diagnosis.

A comparative evaluation of three different preschool vision screening programmes is underway in Newcastle and an initial report was published after 18 months of follow-up.[33] The coverage, identification of target conditions (squints, visual acuity loss) and the test characteristics (sensitivity, specificity and predictive value) were compared between three groups. The first group had their vision checked by orthoptists at 35 months (including Sheridan Gardiner and prism test), the second group had a squint check at 30–36 months (CMOs, HVs (health visitors), GPs), and the third group were asked to 'pick up a thread' at 30 months (HVs). Coverage rates were between 60% and 80%. The prevalence of treated target conditions was significantly higher in the group screened by orthoptists, particularly for the detection of children with visual loss not associated with a squint. The sensitivity was also significantly higher in this group (100%) with only a slight drop in specificity (98%). The positive predictive value in the group screened by orthoptists was 74%.

SCREENING FOR VISUAL IMPAIRMENT OUTSIDE THE UK

Health services in other countries are also reviewing vision testing and several are advocating the continuation and development of screening programmes.

In the USA only about 20% of children are screened for visual problems before school entry.[34] A policy statement by the American Academy of Ophthalmology recommended that all preschool children should be screened when newborn, between 3 and 6 months and at 3–4 years of age. Authors recognize that many questions remain unanswered about the history, detection and treatment of visual disorder but conclude that standardized screening should be incorporated into well-child examinations.[35]

Vision testing at 3 years of age is considered to be an efficient and inexpensive method of screening for visual disorders in Japan. Following a pilot study, testing was incorporated into existing health checks in 1989.[36]

In Denmark an epidemiological study of amblyopia compared the prevalence in an unscreened older population with that in the younger screened population.[37] The prevalence in children today is 1% compared with 2.9% in adults and the authors suggest that this difference is the result of successful screening and treatment. A study in Sweden concluded that population screening at 4 years of age leads to the detection and successful treatment of most cases of amblyopia.[38]

FUTURE DEVELOPMENTS

Strabismus and amblyopia are associated with significant hypermetropia in infancy, and refractive screening in infancy may identify children at increased risk and facilitate close monitoring and early treatment. Photorefraction was developed to assess visual disorders but a refractive screening programme at 6–9 months of age is being evaluated in Cambridge and Avon.[39] The programme has a high capital cost but the equipment can be used by technicians. The screening programme is linked to a controlled trial of spectacle correction of refractive error and should improve understanding of the aetiology and natural history of visual problems in children. Initial results suggest that screening infants is effective, that hypermetropia is a good predictor of strabismus and reduced acuity and that early spectacle correction significantly reduces the incidence of these deficits in later years.[9] The forced preferential looking procedure has also been used to test visual acuity in infants but there is considerable overlap in results obtained from the normal and 'abnormal' populations. This method is more time-consuming and appears to be less sensitive than photorefraction.[3,9]

The Sonksen picture test has been designed to screen binocular vision in children from 21 months of age. It is simple to administer and takes about 2 minutes to complete. Hodes et al[40] estimated the sensitivity of the test to be 65% and specificity to be 47%.

Following the calculation of age-related reference ranges for visual acuity, two alternatives have been proposed which would maintain a 10% screening failure rate.[8] The first is to change the letter sizes according to the age of the child and the second, and probably simplest, is to use the standard letter size but to change the chart distance. This method would allow testing of children who do not present for screening at an exact age.

SUMMARY

Visual deficit is a common problem and early detection and treatment has long been regarded as worthwhile. There are, however, fundamental areas of uncertainty about the normal development of vision and the natural history of visual defects and there remains debate about the benefits of early treatment and its effect on clinical outcome.

Screening does detect some children with visual problems who would not otherwise be identified and, in well-trained hands, the test characteristics can be maintained at a high level. In the absence of screening, 'straight-eyed' amblyopes in particular are seldom detected until they reach school although, even with screening, many escape detection. The age of identification may fall with the increasing use of crowded card systems.

For any screening programme to be successful, it must be readily available to the target population and high coverage must be maintained. Reported coverage rates for the vision screening programmes range from 50% to 95%. There is an inevitable trade-off between the sensitivity and specificity of different screening programmes. Orthoptists generally achieve lower false positive and false negative rates than other health professionals but coverage tends to be lower.[3,29,30,33] Lower coverage in effect decreases the sensitivity of the whole programme. Referral of normal children is costly for the health service and generates parental anxiety while false reassurance of children with problems has obvious costs to the individuals.

Many questions remain unanswered but, if preschool screening for visual defects is to be continued, the effectiveness and efficiency of the programme must be monitored, bearing in mind the costs to individuals, to the community and to the health service. Similarly, new methods of screening should only be introduced after careful evaluation.

KEY POINTS FOR CLINICAL PRACTICE

- Severe visual impairment is uncommon (prevalence 3–4 per 10 000 births) and is usually identified without screening.
- Squint, refractive errors and amblyopia are common, occurring in up to 5% of children.
- The natural history of normal and abnormal visual development remains poorly understood.
- Visual acuity develops gradually and up to 40% of 3-year-olds may not have reached adult levels of acuity for a linear display although many will demonstrate 6/6 acuity for single-letter targets.
- There are few well-designed studies demonstrating that the early treatment of amblyopia results in long-term improvement. However, it is generally believed that treatment is effective and that a trial of conservative management would be unethical.
- The effectiveness and efficiency of any screening programme should be regularly monitored.

REFERENCES

1 Hall DMB, ed. Health for all children. Oxford: Oxford University Press, 1989
2 Hall DMB, ed. Health for all children, 2nd edn. Oxford: Oxford University Press, 1991
3 Bishop AM. Vision screening of children: a review of methods and personnel involved in the UK. Ophthalmic Physiol Opt 1991; 11: 3–9
4 Stewart-Brown SL, Haslum MN, Howlett B. Preschool vision screening: a service in need of rationalisation. Arch Dis Child 1988; 63: 356–359
5 Atkinson J, Braddick O. The development of visual function. In: Davis JA, Dobbing J (eds). Scientific foundations of paediatrics. London: Heinemann, 1981, pp 865–877
6 Atkinson J. Human visual development over the first six months of life. A review and a hypothesis. Hum Neurobiol 1984; 3: 61–74
7 Sonksen PM. The assessment of vision in the preschool child. Arch Dis Child 1993; 68: 513–516
8 Wade AM, Ades AE, Salt AT, Jayatunga R, Sonksen PM. Age-related standards for ordinal data: modelling the changes in visual acuity from 2–9 years of age. Statist Med 1994 (in press)
9 Atkinson J. New tests of vision screening and assessment in infants and young children. In: French JH, Havel S, Casaer P (eds). Child neurology and developmental disabilities. Baltimore: Brookes Publishing, 1989, pp 219–227
10 Ingram RM, Holland WW, Walker C et al. Screening for visual defects in preschool children. Br J Ophthalmol 1986; 70: 16–21
11 Peckham CS. Vision in childhood. Br Med Bull 1986; 42: 150–154
12 Hall DB, Hall SM. Early detection of vision defects in infancy. Br Med J 1988; 296: 823–824
13 Hall SM, Pugh AG, Hall DM. Vision screening in the under 5s. Br Med J 1982; 285: 1096–1098
14 Hall DBM. The child with a handicap. Oxford: Blackwell Scientific, 1984
15 Egan DF, Brown R. Vision testing of young children in the age range 18 months to 4 years. Child Care Health Dev 1984; 10: 381–390
16 Stewart-Brown S. Visual defects in school children: screening policy and education implications. In: Macfarlane JA, ed. Progress in child health. Edinburgh: Churchill Livingstone, 1987: vol 3, pp 14–37
17 Stewart-Brown S, Haslum NH, Butler N. Educational attainment of 10 year old children with treated and untreated visual defects. Devel Med Child Neurol 1985; 27: 504–573
18 Fielder AR. The management of squint. Arch Dis Child 1989; 64: 413–418
19 Harcourt RB. Detection and management of squint. Arch Dis Child 1983; 58: 675–676
20 Ingram RM. The problem of screening children for visual defects. Br J Ophthalmol 1977; 61: 4–7
21 Thompson JR, Woodruff G, Hiscox FA et al. The incidence and prevalence of amblyopia detected in childhood. Public Health 1991; 105: 455–462
22 Ingram RM. Amblyopia. Br Med J 1989; 20: 204
23 Shaw DE, Fielder AR, Minshull C, Rosenthal AR. Amblyopia – factors influencing age of presentation. Lancet 1988; 2: 207–209
24 Hilton AF, Stanley JC. Pitfalls in testing children's vision by the Sheridan Gardiner single optotype method. Br J Ophthalmol 1972; 56: 135–139
25 Taylor D. Screening for squint and poor vision. Arch Dis Child 1987; 62: 982–983
26 Ingram RM, Holland WW, Walker C, Wilson JM, Arnold PE, Dally S. A first attempt to prevent amblyopia and squint by spectacle correction of abnormal refractions from age 1 year. Br J Ophthalmol 1985; 69: 851–853
27 Wormald RP. Preschool vision screening in Cornwall: performance indicators of community orthoptists. Arch Dis Child 1991; 66: 917–920
28 Allen J, Bose B. An audit of preschool vision screening. Arch Dis Child 1992; 67: 1292–1293
29 Bolger PG, Stewart-Brown SL, Newcombe E, Starbuck A. Vision screening in preschool children: comparison of orthoptists and clinical medical officers as primary screeners. Br Med J 1991; 303: 1291–1294
30 Stayte M, Wortham C, Reeves B. Orthoptists reduce false positive hospital referrals. Health Trends 1992; 24(4): 157–160

31 Feldman WM, Milner RA, Sackett B, Gilbert S. Effects of preschool screening for vision and hearing on the prevalence of vision and hearing problems 6–12 months later. Lancet 1980; 2: 1014–1016

32 Rona RJ, Reynolds A, Allsop M et al. Audit from preschool developmental surveillance of vision, hearing and language referrals. Arch Dis Child 1991; 66: 921–926

33 Jarvis SN, Tamhne RC, Thompson L et al. Preschool vision screening. Arch Dis Child 1990; 65: 288–294

34 Essman SW, Essman TF. Screening for pediatric eye disease. Am Fam Physician 1992; 46: 1243–1252

35 Fulton A. Screening preschool children to detect visual and ocular disorders. Arch Ophthalmol 1992; 110: 1553–1554

36 Yazawa K, Suga J, Wakita S et al. The Tokyo home vision screening program for amblyopia in 3 year old children. Am J Ophthalmol 1992; 114: 416–419

37 Vinding T, Gregerson E, Jensen A, Rindziunski E. Prevalence of amblyopia in old people without previous screening and treatment. An evaluation of the present prophylactic procedures among children in Denmark. Acta Ophthalmol (Copenh) 1991; 69: 796–798

38 Sjostrand J, Abrahamsson M. Risk factors in amblyopia. Eye 1990; 4: 787–793

39 Atkinson J. Assessment of vision in infants and young children. In: Harel S, Anastasiow NJ, eds. The at risk infant: psycho/social/medical aspects. Baltimore: Brookes Publishing, 1985, pp 341–352

40 Hodes DT, Sonksen PM, McKee M. Evaluation of the Sonksen picture test for detection of minor visual problems in the surveillance of preschool children. Dev Med Child. Neurol 1994; 36: 16–25

7. New thoughts on the management of behavioural problems in preschool children

P. Stallard

PREVALENCE AND SIGNIFICANCE

Community surveys have consistently found high rates of significant behavioural problems in preschool children. In a survey of 705 3-year-old children living in the London borough of Waltham Forest, 7% were found to have marked problems and a further 15% mild problems.[1] Similar rates have been found in inner city and more rural areas,[2,3] in children of West Indian born parents living in London, Asian born parents living in Birmingham,[4,5] and in community studies conducted in America and Canada.[6-8] The adoption of a definition which includes both marked and moderate problems would therefore indicate that at any one time approximately 20% of preschool children are displaying difficult and concerning behaviour.

The frequency of individual behaviours varies, although nocturnal enuresis, sleeping, eating and general management problems occur comparatively often. Almost one-third of 3-year-old children are in nappies or wet the bed at least three nights per week. One-quarter either regularly sleep in their parents' bed, wake at night or take over an hour to settle at bedtime. Approximately one in ten is either extremely faddy with their eating or considered by their parents to nearly always have a small appetite, with slightly fewer finding their child to be frequently difficult to control. Other behaviours are comparatively less common with between 1% and 4% of children being considered by their parents to be frequently miserable or to have many worries.[1,3]

The behaviour of girls and boys is not significantly different although boys have a tendency to be more active and girls more fearful.[1,3,6] Birth order does, however, affect how parents perceive their child, with parents of only children having significantly more concerns about their child's behaviour even though they behave no differently from those with siblings.[3]

CONTINUITY

There is substantive evidence to demonstrate that behavioural difficulties are not short-lived and tend to persist over time.[9,10] In the Waltham Forest study a sample of children were followed-up and assessed at age 4 and age 8. Of those children who displayed behavioural problems at age 3, 63% continued to display difficulties when assessed 12 months later and 62% presented with difficulties of at least mild, moderate, or severe level at age 8. This compared with only 11% and 22% of the control group at age 4 and age 8 respectively.[1]

The child's sex was a significant predictor of outcome with 73% of males in the problem group continuing to display difficult behaviour at age 8 compared to 43% of females. The severity of the behaviour was also important with almost three-quarters of those 3-year-olds with severe or moderate difficulties continuing to show problems 5 years later. There was also some evidence to suggest a similarity between the types of problem presented by the children at different ages. Fearful 3-year-olds were more likely to show emotional problems whereas overactive children were more likely to show conduct disorders.

FAMILY FACTORS

Significant relationships between the presence of behavioural problems, adverse maternal mental health and family functioning have been found.[11] Approximately 30% of mothers with young children present with depressive symptoms.[1] Depressed mothers have been found to be more likely to report poor relationships with their own parents, marry early and have their first child before the age of 21.[12] They tend to be alone with their child for the majority of the day although they are not particularly socially isolated, often having relatives or friends nearby.[12] Poor quality of marriage marked by high rates of partner conflict, constant quarrelling and a lack of cooperation are also associated with behavioural problems.[1,12]

Examination of the interactions between mothers and their children has found that depressed mothers are less effective and able to sensitively and appropriately respond to their child's behaviour. They make fewer reciprocal responses towards their child during joint activities and the child fails to respond to more of their mother's responses.[13]

THE IDENTIFICATION OF BEHAVIOURAL PROBLEMS

Despite the prevalence and significance of such problems, comparatively few preschool children with behavioural problems are referred to the specialist secondary services. The personal view of one GP was that for 'each child referred to child-guidance clinics there are five equally disturbed not referred'.[14] This view is consistent with the findings of a recent study where only one in eight of those parents who expressed a lot of concern about one or more aspects of their child's behaviour was referred to the multidisciplinary child and family mental health service.[15] Obviously, referrals to specialist mental health services do not reflect identification rates. In a number of instances behavioural problems may be identified, although some families may not want a referral feeling that this will be a sign of personal inadequacy, failure, or stigmatizing. Others may receive help from other child-focused professionals, particularly health visitors who are one of the few professional groups who have regular contact with preschool children and their families in their home environment. Nevertheless, it does question how many preschool behavioural problems are correctly identified.

A study in general practice found that only 2% of parents specifically consulted their GP about preschool behavioural or management problems. Medical concerns were frequently presented as the reason for consultation although these often disguised behavioural problems which the GP rarely succeeded in identifying.[16] Similarly, a survey of parents whose child was referred to a specialist behaviour management service found that none had considered going to their GP for advice about behavioural problems.[17]

Many of the complaints presented to medical staff have been found to have a substantial behavioural or emotional component. Of 3- and 4-year-old children attending general and surgical paediatric outpatient clinics 50% and 39% respectively have been found to have significant behavioural problems.[18] Similar findings have been reported by those examining school-aged children.

Mental health problems have been found to be present in between 23% and 28% of those attending general practice and paediatric outpatient clinics although once again many of these go unrecognized.[19,20] It is therefore probable that a large number of preschool behavioural problems remain unidentified.

The routine assessment of preschool children in order to identify those displaying or at risk of developing behavioural problems would therefore appear to be an important objective of child health services.

THE ROUTINE ASSESSMENT OF PRESCHOOL BEHAVIOUR

The Association of Child Psychologists and Psychiatrists in conjunction with the Health Visitors Association has highlighted the central role of the health visitor in the prevention, identification, assessment and treatment of preschool behavioural problems.[21] The report recommended that the behaviour of preschool children should be routinely assessed using parent-completed checklists and that these should be incorporated into child health surveillance programmes.

Assessment considerations

The routine use of behaviour checklists needs to address three issues:[22]

1. The amount of time available to conduct such assessments is limited and therefore any checklist must be quick to administer and easy to complete.
2. The reliability and validity of any assessment should be assessed since the screening efficiency of many checklists is poor.

3. The checklist must take account of the parents' views regarding the child's behaviour.

This last point is especially important — highlighting a fundamental difficulty in this area, namely that of definition. There is no universal agreement about what is a problem behaviour since parents will view the same behaviour differently. This perception is often influenced by their own previous experiences, expectations and practical circumstances. Parental perception is therefore important and will be an indication for the clinician as to what form of intervention is required.

The Behaviour Checklist

There are comparatively few assessments specifically designed to assess the behaviour of preschool children. At nurseries and playgroups the Preschool Behaviour Questionnaire has been used although this questionnaire is completed by nursery staff and does not contain any questions relating to night-times or mealtimes.[23] In home settings, the Behaviour Screening Questionnaire (BSQ) is one of the most commonly used and has been found to correctly identify 90% of children attending a psychiatric clinic.[24] However, the BSQ is professionally completed, takes approximately 30 minutes to complete and does not include an assessment of the parents' view. A parent-completed derivative of this, the Behaviour Checklist (BCL), has been developed which can be used as a screening instrument to practically identify behavioural problems.[25] The BCL consists of 21 questions covering the general areas of eating, sleeping, soiling, wetting, speech, activity level, concentration, dependency, control/management, temper tantrums, mood, worries, fearfulness, and relationships with both peers and siblings. The checklist takes only a few minutes to complete with the parent choosing which of three or four descriptions best describes their child's behaviour over the previous 4 weeks. For the purpose of scoring, those questions relating to wetting and speech are omitted since at this age they are more an indication of development rather than of behavioural problems. The remaining 17 items are scored 0, 1, or 2 according to severity, and, in order to avoid undue emphasis upon any one area in which there is more than one question, the highest rating is used to determine the total score for that particular area. A cut-off score of 10 has been found to correctly identify 82% of those children with severe and moderate problems detected by the BSQ. This included a false positive rate of 12.6% and a false negative rate of 30.4%.[25]

Parental perception

In a clinical context the use of such symptom-loading methods to identify children with behavioural problems poses three major problems.

First, reliance on aggregated scores fails to identify those children displaying only one or two behaviours which are nonetheless causing their parents significant difficulty. Their total score would be below the cut-off criteria and they would not be identified as experiencing difficulties.

Secondly, there is an assumed relationship between the description of a child's behaviour and the presence of a problem. For example, there is an assumption that a child who frequently sleeps in their parents' bed is a problem, although a recent study found that of the 12% of children who regularly slept in their parents' bed only 2% of parents expressed a lot of concern about this.[3] A number of parents did not therefore view it as a problem, with some identifying a number of positive reasons for wishing this to happen.

Finally, focusing on overall scores fails to identify lesser concerns which could be addressed at an early stage. The inclusion of a rating of parental concern could alert screeners to lesser, although real, worries so that it could be used in a more preventive manner.

BEHAVIOURAL ASSESSMENT IN PRACTICE

Despite the potential value of the BCL in the assessment of preschool behaviour, few studies have reported its use. One reported the development of a multiple criteria screen to identify families in the community where the mothers and/or their toddlers were experiencing psychological difficulties. Health visitors assessed maternal mental health and the behaviour of preschool children using both standardized measures and a health visitor questionnaire. A total of 55% of the sample were identified as experiencing problems. The actual number of children identified by the use of the BCL was not specified although the authors concluded that the screen was efficient and acceptable to families.[26]

The routine assessment of behaviour using the BCL, modified to include a rating of parental concern, has become a standard part of the 3-year-old developmental check undertaken in Bath Health District. After parents have described their child's behaviour, they are asked to indicate their degree of concern, rating this on a three-point scale. The BCL is then used as a brief semistructured interview conducted by health visitors designed to gain an overview of the child, highlighting both positive behaviours and those identified by parents as being of concern.

All health visitors participate in a week-long course designed to train them in the administration of the district developmental screening programme. One session is devoted to understanding the significance of behaviour problems, familiarization with the BCL and practice in facilitating its completion. The results of a sample of 1170 BCLs completed during 1990 revealed that 16% of parents expressed a lot of concern about one or more aspects of their child's behaviour, with a further 50% expressing slight concerns. A breakdown of parental concern relating to the various behaviours included in the BCL is presented in Table 7.1.

Table 7.1 Prevalence (%) of individual behaviours rated as definitely present on the BCL and degree of parental concern ($n = 1170$)

BCL item	Definitely present	A lot of concern	Slightly concerned	Not at all concerned
Poor appetite	8	4	22	74
Faddy eating	11	3	18	79
Night-time wetting	31	1	9	90
Daytime wetting	6	1	5	94
Soiling	5	2	4	94
Night-time settling	7	3	14	83
Night-time waking	10	3	17	80
Sleeps in parents' bed	12	2	12	86
Overactive	8	2	9	89
Poor concentration	5	1	7	92
Clingy	3	1	10	89
Demands attention	4	2	11	87
Difficult to control	7	5	22	73
Tantrums	5	3	17	80
Unhappy mood	2	1	6	93
Worrier	3	1	7	92
Fearful	1	1	8	91
Poor sibling relationship	0.5	1	6	93
Poor peer relationship	1	1	8	91

Feedback from both health visitors and parents about the BCL has been extremely positive. Health visitors have found it a useful way of structuring interviews by providing a framework which covers all aspects of the child's behaviour. This in turn enables more focused contact by clearly highlighting and agreeing with parents those problems which will form the basis of interventions. It enables lesser, although nonetheless real, concerns to be addressed in a more preventive manner by discussing them at an early stage. Most importantly, the BCL provides an opportunity to reinforce positive parenting, good aspects of the child's behaviour and a chance to constructively challenge parental doubts regarding the adequacy of their parenting. Being a parent is a task for which many parents feel poorly prepared and is often characterized by feelings of self-doubt, criticism, and inadequacy. The opportunity to reinforce parental practice has been commented upon by some health visitors who have felt that parents had become more positive and confident in their interactions with their child following this assessment.

Parents have been similarly positive, with a number welcoming the opportunity to talk about their child. Indeed, parents have few opportunities to routinely discuss their child's behaviour, often feeling that they need a significant problem before troubling busy professionals. Typically such contacts are parent-initiated, problem-focused, and usually result in the most pressing problem being discussed whilst others remain neglected. The provision of an opportunity to discuss all aspects of their child has been valued by parents who have reported feeling freer to talk about other lesser worries. However, in order to achieve such open discussion parents require a clear explanation as to the purpose of the BCL and reassurance that it is not solely to identify problems.

THE MANAGEMENT OF BEHAVIOURAL PROBLEMS

The results of these and other studies would suggest that the routine assessment of preschool children will identify large numbers with problem or concerning behaviour.[3,22,26] Whilst some of these parents may not want any intervention, it is probable that the demand for services will be high and will place particular demands upon community services. It is therefore important to consider what frontline interventions are available to community services and how limited secondary services can be organized in a flexible and accessible manner that provides their specialist skills to maximum effect.

Frontline management

There are a variety of frontline interventions available for the management of behaviour problems. Some require knowledge about specific treatment interventions whereas others relate to the non-specific effects of contact with a helping professional. Parents find the opportunity to talk and be understood as one of the most helpful aspects of intervention, often more helpful than the actual treatment techniques themselves.[17,27] In terms of non-specific factors, the following would seem worthy of consideration by practitioners.

Validation

The process of validation is important and yet is often overlooked by many professionals. It provides an opportunity to confirm a parent's situation, acknowledge how they are feeling and understand why they have chosen, or been forced, to respond to their child's behaviour in such a manner. The vast majority of parents are well intentioned and do not deliberately or consciously set out to mismanage or create problems. This needs to be acknowledged and their method of management validated rather than be subjected to professional criticism.

Validation requires non-judgemental listening and acceptance of parents' experiences. Possible reasons for the current difficulties other than individual failure should be highlighted. Some parents, for example, may take a child into their bed for comfort when ill and this may then become a learned routine resulting in the child being reluctant to return to their own bed when well. The parent has acted in a caring and understandable manner and the subsequent problem is due to inappropriate learning rather than personal failure or inadequacy.

Reassurance

Parents regularly find themselves confronted with situations in which they have to make immediate decisions regarding the management of their child's behaviour. A number regularly question their decisions and would undoubtedly welcome the opportunity to discuss such issues in an informal way with an informed person. This appears to be especially true of first-time parents who have been found to be more concerned about their child's behaviour.[3]

On other occasions parents may need reassurance that their method of dealing with their child's behaviour is effective and may require encouragement to continue. Indeed, the introduction of new methods of management often results in an initial worsening of the child's behaviour and may be interpreted by parents as an indication of ineffectiveness.[28] An awareness of this possibility and professional reassurance during this initial stage can be a useful intervention. However, it is important that the situation continues to be monitored so that parents are not given a false sense of security. If improvements are not forthcoming alternative interventions may be required.

Positive empowerment

Parents are often good at highlighting their inadequacies and failures rather than acknowledging their success. Consultations with professionals are often problem-based, thereby reinforcing parents' negative perception of their abilities. It is therefore essential to provide a more balanced perspective by both acknowledging problems and highlighting positive aspects of the child's behaviour. The importance of such an empowering approach should not be underestimated since some contacts with professionals have been found to undermine confidence, reduce parental self-esteem and increase dependency upon outside agencies.[29]

The process of empowerment involves highlighting and building upon parental strengths and skills in order to help parents understand their child's behaviour and decide upon a course of management. It should be emphasized that there are often no quick or easy solutions since such a simplistic approach is undermining parental resources and confidence. The working model is one of partnership whereby professionals work with parents to help them problem-solve rather than providing answers and advice. This in turn empowers parents, demonstrates that they can find solutions to their difficulties and increases their commitment to succeed. In many situations parents know what to do but for whatever reason feel unable to act in such a manner. Attempts to tell parents what to do are typically met with failure or, if they are successful, result in the parents becoming increasingly dependent upon outside professionals to resolve their problems.

Education and the provision of information

There is evidence that the general provision of information regarding potential behavioural problems may not be helpful. In one study, the parents of children assessed at 9 months and 2 years of age who received regular health visiting and preparatory information leaflets reported more problems with their child's behaviour than a control group who received no anticipatory guidance.[30] Parents may have become preoccupied with their child's behaviour, resulting in them becoming more aware of potential problems.

Whilst anticipatory guidance might sensitize parents to their child's future behaviour, a number of parents will currently be experiencing problems with which they would like help. Preparation for parenthood is non-existent, with parents often finding themselves in a position whereby they are assumed to have the relevant knowledge to understand and effectively manage their child's behaviour. Levels of knowledge are variable, expectations often high, resulting in some parents labouring under misapprehensions about how their child should behave. The provision of information as to typical toddler behaviour is sometimes enough to put a parental concern in perspective and help the parent realize that their child's behaviour is similar to that of others. Information as to the frequency of nocturnal enuresis and the natural progression over time can help some parents understand that their child's bed wetting is not so unusual. This may result in it becoming less of a concern for the parents and less of an issue for the child. Similarly, an information leaflet for parents who reported sleep problems was found to result in 43% of identified sleep problems improving without any further intervention.[31]

Interventions

Assessment

A number of studies have reported the use of behavioural interventions by a range of professionals. These interventions require a detailed assessment of the child's behaviour, particularly the antecedents that precede it, the consequences that follow and a clear description of the behaviour itself. The success of any subsequent programme will largely depend upon an accurate and thorough assessment. However, the assessment process itself can be very positive and result in changes in parenting practice or perception that negate the need for further intervention.[32] A behaviour diary, recording both the day and time of the behaviour, what was happening, what the child did, and the consequences that followed is an extremely useful tool for the practitioner. This provides information on frequency and behaviour patterns which can guide the family into devising an effective management programme.

Behavioural interventions

Behavioural interventions have focused upon a variety of specific behavioural problems including sleeping difficulties,[33] infant crying,[34] feeding and failure to thrive,[35] and constipation,[36] whereas others have focused upon general behavioural problems.[17,37] They have been delivered by clinical nurse specialists,[17] specialist health visitors,[38] and community health visitors, jointly with either clinical psychologists,[39] child psychiatrists[33,37] or with other teams of professionals.[35] These interventions have been provided either in groups[40] or individually,[41] in home[17] and in clinic settings.[31]

The effectiveness of these interventions has varied, with a number demonstrating significant reductions in problem behaviour[27,39,41] and high rates of consumer satisfaction.[17] Others have failed to demonstrate that behavioural interventions delivered by health visitors result in significant improvements.[21,31,33] The reasons for this are at present unclear although inadequate training in behavioural interventions and the effectiveness of such methods with well-established problems have been discussed. A recent review concluded that behavioural interventions are particularly effective for mild behavioural problems of short duration where the family is relatively stable. They are less effective when problems are extensive, well established and occur with other or multiple difficulties.[28] In such situations they should be referred to the secondary services.

Monitoring

In some instances perceptions of a child's behaviour may differ, resulting in professional concern not being shared by the family. Unless there is a shared view and the family is motivated and able to explore alternative methods of management it is extremely unlikely that any positive change will occur. These situations are common and difficult for professionals who feel frustrated and powerless and often interpret this lack of change as their own personal failure or inadequacy. Being clear as to the goal of contact is essential since understanding that the purpose of visiting is to monitor rather than actively change is professionally quite freeing.[42] In such situations professionals have a responsibility to continue to monitor the child's behaviour, help the parents recognize its significance, and in extreme cases a duty to bring it to the attention of the Social Services Department.

The organization of secondary services

Specialist secondary services need to ensure that limited resources are provided in a flexible manner so that their expertise is widely available and accessible to both families and the professionals with whom they have contact. It is therefore important that secondary services provide a range of services.

Liaison

Liaison refers to the partnership between mental health and medical services, secondary and primary care in order to provide an integrated approach to assessment and treatment.[43] The development of such services for preschool children would seem important in view of the large number of children with behaviour problems found to present to medical staff with physical symptoms.[9,16,18] Examples of child psychiatry liasion services with paediatrics have been reported which have identified many benefits.[44,45] In particular, they can result in better assessment and management of individual children, increased awareness of psychological factors in physical illness and improved professional relationships.[43]

The development of a liaison service requires the pro-active establishment of regular links with the paediatric service and community team. It is essentially a service targeted upon staff rather than one provided directly to clients, and in order to be effective requires prompt and clear communications from the child mental health team that are both practical and understandable.[43,45]

Consultation

Consultation has been defined as a 'process involving a consultant who is invited to help a consultee with a work related issue'.[46] In this context it would involve the specialist child mental health team meeting with the professional who already has contact with a family in order to clarify issues, areas of concern and desired outcomes. An action plan is jointly agreed which is then implemented by the involved professional and reviewed with the consultant at an agreed date. The consultation attempts to clarify the key issues for both the worker and the family, the necessity and appropriateness of intervention and the agency or professional best suited to undertake this work. Consultation can occur either individually or in groups and in a regular, planned way or on a case by case basis.

A health visitor consultation service provided by clinical psychologists has identified many benefits to both families and health visitors.[42,47] In particular, consultation acts as a filter, providing health visitors with the necessary clarity and skills to carry on working with a large number of families whilst identifying those with more complex problems which require specialist intervention.

Training

The management of behavioural problems forms a substantial part of a health visitors workload although, in one study, almost half of those surveyed felt that their training did not equip them for this role and virtually all felt that they had a need for further training.[48] Similar findings have been reported by other researchers who have emphasized the need for training in both behaviour therapy and counselling skills.[17,37]

The role of specialist secondary services in providing training is therefore clear, although particular thought needs to be paid to the method by which this occurs. Behavioural training workshops have been found to have a consolidating effect upon clinical practice rather than providing new assessment and treatment skills. The acquisition of new skills may need to occur over a longer period of training involving a supervised training period, regular liaison and in vivo training.[32,49]

Direct referral service

A number of preschool children with behavioural problems will require specialist interventions. Local mental health services need to clarify their role with this age group and consider the development of specific preschool services.[50] Referers need to be educated as to appropriate cases and ensure that referrals are discussed and agreed with parents. Professionals need information about referral procedures, case management, methods of work, service organization and communication. Families need information about the service, what happens during meetings, who will be seen and how many times they will meet. The service needs to be both acceptable and accessible to families and should be provided in a range of settings, including the family's own home, community clinics, paediatric outpatients and GP surgeries.[51,52]

Finally, joint assessments and work with other professionals should be undertaken since these tend to improve working relationships, clarify appropriate referrals, share shills, and result in improvements in assessment and treatment skills.[37,40]

KEY POINTS FOR CLINICAL PRACTICE

- The assessment of preschool behaviour should be routinely undertaken and become an integral part of child health surveillance programmes. The assessment should be parent-completed and include an evaluation of parental perception.
- Professionals should adopt a positive empowering approach, highlighting positive aspects of the child's behaviour, building upon parental skills and strengths, and facilitating problem-solving.
- The non-specific aspects of contact are perceived by parents to be as important as the specific treatment techniques themselves. Important skills involve listening, validation and reassurance.
- The general provision of anticipatory information about behavioural problems may not be helpful. However, for those already experiencing problems information can be reassuring and help parents put their concerns in perspective.
- Behavioural interventions should only be undertaken following a thorough and detailed assessment which should involve some form of record-keeping. The assessment process and be a powerful intervention for some families.

- Behavioural interventions are particularly effective for specific problems of short duration and without significant family disturbance. Complex, multiple problems of long duration associated with significant family and social issues should be referred to the secondary services.
- Secondary services need to clarify their role with preschool children and provide a range of services, including liaison, consultation, training and joint work. The development of a service focusing specifically upon preschool children should be considered.

REFERENCES

1 Richman N, Stevenson JE, Graham PJ. Preschool to school: a behavioural study. London: Academic Press, 1982
2 Jenkins S, Bax M, Hart H. Behaviour problems in preschool children. J Child Psychol Psychiatry 1980; 21: 5–17
3 Stallard P. The behaviour of 3-year-old children: prevalence and parental perception of problem behaviour: a research note. J Child Psychol Psychiatry 1993; 34: 413–421
4 Earls F, Richman N. The prevalence of behaviour problems in three-year old children of West Indian-born parents. J Child Psychol Psychiatry 1980; 21: 99–106
5 Newth SJ, Corbett J. Behaviour and emotional problems in three-year-old children of Asian parentage. J Child Psychol Psychiatry 1993; 34: 333–352
6 Earls F. Prevalence of behaviour problems in 3-year-old children. Arch Gen Psychiatry 1980; 37: 1153–1157
7 Cornely P, Bromet E. Prevalence of behaviour problems in three-year-old children living near Three Mile Island: a comparative analysis. J Child Psychol Psychiatry 1986; 27: 489–498
8 Minde R, Minde K. Behavioural screening of preschool children: a new approach to mental health? In: Graham PJ, ed. Epidemiological approaches in child psychiatry. London: Academic Press, 1977
9 Hart H, Bax M, Jenkins S. Health and behaviour in preschool children. Child Care Health Dev 1984; 10: 1–16
10 Lerner JA, Inui TS, Trupin EW, Douglas E. Preschool behaviour can predict future psychiatric disorders. J Am Acad Child Psychiatry 1985; 25: 42–48
11 Ghodsian M, Zajicek E, Wolkind S. A longitudinal study of maternal depression and child behaviour problems. J Child Psychol Psychiatry 1984; 25: 91–109
12 Pound A, Cox A, Puckering C, Mills M. The impact of depression on young children. In: Stevenson J, ed. Recent research in developmental psychopathology. JCPP book supplement No 4. Oxford: Pergamon Press, 1985
13 Mills M, Puckering C, Pound A, Cox A. What is it about depressed mothers that influences their children's functioning? In: Stevenson J, ed. Recent research in developmental psychopathology. JCPP book supplement No 4. Oxford: Pergamon Press, 1985
14 Ryle A. Psychotherapy by general practitioners. Proc R Soc Med 1963; 56: 834–837
15 Stallard P. Routine assessment of children at three years. Health Visitor 1993; 66: 397–398
16 Bax M, Hart H. Health needs of preschool children. Arch Dis Child 1976; 51: 848–852
17 Pritchard P. Behavioural work with preschool children in the community. Health Visitor 1994; 67: 54–56
18 Fitzgerald M. Behavioural deviance and maternal depressive symptoms in paediatric outpatients. Arch Dis Child 1985; 60: 560–562
19 Garralda ME, Bailey D. Children with psychiatric disorders in primary care. J Child Psychol Psychiatry 1986; 27: 611–624
20 Garralda ME, Bailey D. Psychiatric disorders in general paediatric referrals. Arch Dis Child 1989; 64: 1727–1733

21 Stevenson J. Health visitor based services for preschool children with behaviour problems. Association of Child Psychology and Psychiatry, 1990: Occasional Paper No 2

22 Hewitt K. Assessment by health visitors of behaviour problems in pre-school children. In: Stevenson J, ed. Health visitor based services for preschool children with behaviour problems. Association of Child Psychology and Psychiatry, 1990: Occasional Paper No 2

23 McGuire J, Richman N. The prevalence of behavioural problems in three types of preschool group. J Child Psychol Psychiatry 1986; 27: 455–472

24 Richman N, Graham PJ. A behavioural screening questionnaire for use with 3-year old children. Preliminary findings. J Child Psychol Psychiatry 1971; 12: 5–33

25 Richman N. Is a behaviour checklist for preschool children useful? In: Graham PJ, ed. Epidemiological approaches to child psychiatry. London: Academic Press, 1977

26 Nicol AR, Stretch DD, Fundudis T, Smith I, Davison I. The nature of mother and toddler problems 1. Development of a multiple criteria screen. J Child Psychol Psychiatry 1987; 28: 739–754

27 Galbraith L, Hewitt KE, Pritchard L. Behavioural treatment for sleep disturbance. Health Visitor 1993; 66: 169–171

28 McAuley R. Counselling parents in child behaviour therapy. Arch Dis Child 1992; 67: 536–542

29 Clements J. Update — training parents of mentally handicapped children. Assoc Child Psychol Psychiatry News 1985; 7: 2–9

30 Hewitt K, Mason L, Snelson W, Crawford W. Parent education in preventing behaviour problems. Health Visitor 1991; 64: 415–417

31 Richards E, Bidder RT, Gardner S. Sleep clinics with health visitors: a 2-year evaluation. Child Care Health Dev 1992; 18: 395–404

32 Appleton P. Interventions by health visitors. In: Stevenson J, ed. Health visitor based services for preschool children with behaviour problems. Association of Child Psychology and Psychiatry, 1990: Occasional Paper No 2

33 Weir IK, Dinnick S. Behaviour modification in the treatment of sleep problems occurring in young children: a controlled trial using health visitors as therapists. Child Care Health Dev 1988; 14: 355–367

34 Pritchard P. An infant crying clinic. Health Visitor 1986; 59: 375–377

35 Iwaniec D, Herbert M, McNeish A. Social work with failure-to-thrive children and their families. 11: Behavioural social work intervention. Br J Soc Work 1985; 15: 375–389

36 Almond P. A family-centred approach. Health Visitor 1993; 66: 404–405

37 Thompson MJJ, Bellenis C. A joint assessment and treatment service for the under fives. Assoc Child Psychol Psychiatry Newsl 1992; 14: 221–227

38 Roberts S. Tackling sleep problems through a clinic-based approach. Health Visitor 1993; 66: 173–174

39 Carpenter A. Sleep problems: a group approach. Health Visitor 1990; 63: 305–307

40 Szyndler J, Bell G. Are groups for parents of children with sleep problems effective? Health Visitor 1992; 65: 277–279

41 Bellenis C, Thompson MJJ. A joint assessment and treatment service for the under fives — work with health visitors in a child guidance clinic. Part 2. Work done and outcome. Assoc Child Psychol Psychiatry Newsl 1992; 14: 262–266

42 Stallard P. Consultation service relieves the pressure. Prof Care Mother Child 1991; 1: 105–106

43 Black D, McFadyen A, Broster G. Development of a liaison service. Arch Dis Child 1990; 65: 1373–1375

44 McFadyen A, Broster G, Black D. The impact of a child psychiatry liaison service on patterns of referral. Br J Psychiatry 1991; 158: 93–96

45 Leslie SA. Paediatric liaison. Arch Dis Child 1992; 67: 1046–1049

46 Ovretveit J, Brunning H, Huffington C. Adapt or decay: why clinical psychologists must develop the consulting role. Clin Psychol Forum 1992; 46: 27–29

47 Stallard P. The development and evaluation of a health visitor consultation service. Clin Psychol Forum 1991; 35: 10–12

48 Fundudis T. A survey of health visitors' views on the relevance of behavioural techniques for their case work. In: Stevenson J, ed. Health visitor based services for preschool children with behaviour problems. Association of Child Psychology and Psychiatry, 1990: Occasional Paper No 2

49 Hewitt K, Hobday A, Crawford W. What do health visitors gain from behavioural workshops? Child Care Health Dev 1989; 15: 265–275
50 Beer R. A preschool child psychiatric service: referral patterns and service uptake. Child Care Health Dev 1991; 17: 337–355
51 Subotsky F, Brown RMA. Working alongside the general practitioner: a child psychiatric clinic in the general practice setting. Child Care Health Dev 1990; 16: 189–196
52 Vas Dias S, McKenzie SA. Paediatric psychotherapy: a service in a general outpatient clinic. Arch Dis Child 1992; 67: 132–134

8. Early childhood development — education/health interface

T. David

When one of the great world pioneers of nursery education, Margaret McMillan, began her work in Bradford and Deptford in the early part of this century, one of her principal aims was the improvement of children's health through links with the health professions, support for parents in need, and sound education concerning health for the children. Almost a century later, I cannot better these as the main foci for this chapter. I intend to consider the issues which arise from:

1. Holistic services for young children and their families
2. Health and safety implications in early childhood settings
3. Health education in early childhood
4. Health surveillance by teachers and other early childhood educators
5. Interprofessional collaboration and training.

HOLISTIC SERVICES FOR YOUNG CHILDREN: THE EDUCATION/CARE DEBATE

In order to set the idea of holistic services for young children in context, it is necessary to explain, briefly, where our youngest children (ages 0–8 years) are to be found.

As a result of the historical development of nursery education alongside care facilities in the public sector (for 'rescue'), those in the private sector (for working parents), and those in the voluntary sector (largely a result of the shortfall in nursery education), there has been a long and difficult divide in the UK between services deemed 'care' and those deemed 'educational'.[1] However, a recently formed Early Childhood Education Forum (ECEF), bringing together representatives from the many different non-governmental organizations involved in early years provision, and linked by the National Children's Bureau Early Childhood Unit, is aimed at presenting 'one voice'. The ECEF members believe that the care and education of the young child should be holistic, that the two are inseparable, and that wherever young children are to be cared for they should be entitled to appropriate learning opportunities — education.

No British Government to date has implemented a national policy of provision for the under-fives, so that, compared with their counterparts in

109

most countries of the European Union, the parents of children aged under 5 years in Britain have grave difficulties in procuring access to publicly funded daycare, and only 26% of 3- and 4-year-olds are enabled to attend nursery groups provided under the education service.[2-4]

Much of the shortfall for those parents wanting group experiences for their children before they begin formal primary schooling is currently made up by playgroups. These are usually sessional, part-time settings run in non-purpose-built premises, by volunteers and low-paid workers, who have a basic training. For those parents needing daycare while they go out to work, many new, fee-paying day nurseries have sprung up recently, but they may employ staff who are relatively untrained, despite the fact that the Children Act 1989 and the guidelines which followed were intended to raise standards relating to both premises and staffing.

The picture we have then, is that most under-threes are looked after in their own or a relative's or childminder's home. A small number of babies and toddlers attend social services or private daycare facilities.

Meanwhile most 3-year-olds are either attending a playgroup for a few sessions a week while being looked after by their own family or a childminder, or attending a private or maintained nursery.

Four-year-olds are largely attending playgroups and maintained nurseries on a part-time basis until they are (generally) admitted to a primary school reception class in the September of the academic year in which they will become 5. Attendance in such a class before the age of 5 years is attained may be part-time or full-time depending on the policy of the school and the child's ability to cope with the full school day. In addition, a small number of schools have begun to offer out-of-hours care for children of working parents.

The majority of older children, those aged 4–8 years, attend primary schools, where the National Curriculum is legally enforcible in classes for children aged 5–16. In fact, the education reforms are having both positive and negative influences on the experiences of 4-year-olds in the reception classes of primary schools and of children in under-fives settings: the positive being the increased interest in learning and under-fives, the negative being that in many cases teaching approaches and pressure from outside the schools have not taken account of the learning styles and needs of children in this age range.

It is not possible here to provide a full description of the range of facilities for young children in the care/education sector, but it must be acknowledged that there have been some attempts to synthesize the most appropriate elements of daycare and education in the small number of family, or combined, centres opened by some local authorities administered jointly by local social and education services.

The issues arising from this confusion and fragmentation of services for very young children in the UK are many and various.

For parents and their children the main issues are, first, the unequal access, dependent as this is on what exists locally. Despite the present Government's insistence on the retention of the private and voluntary sectors as markers of choice in a market economy, the reality is that most parents have no choice whatsoever.[4] In particular, the lack of provision for children under 3 is a crucial issue for parents. Secondly, most parents do not understand the different types of provision, often using the global, hybrid term 'playschool', from which one can tell little about the form of provision without asking further questions, such as 'Do you pay any fees?', etc. The publication of local data, following the Children Act's triennial reviews, is indeed an improvement on the haphazard information available for parents in the past. Thirdly, the learning opportunities offered children in different types of settings may vary widely, as do the qualifications, pay and conditions of staff.

For colleagues from other services, the issues relating to educational services for young children centre upon the lack of a coherent national policy, and the confusion and fragmentation which results from the different forms of provision. This can frequently result in problems with liaison, collaboration and cooperation. Further, there are different approaches and expectations because of the differing levels of training and attitudes towards professionalization.

For the early years teachers and other educators themselves, the issues revolve around the low status of the work, unclear central policy and, sometimes, local policy, the need for a coherent system of initial and continuing education and training to work with young children, including a degree-level route for those wishing to specialize in provision for the nought-to-threes. At least at continuing professional development level there should be opportunities to undertake multiprofessional training, to engage with colleagues from the health and other fields, in order to provide holistic services for young children and their families acknowledging and respecting the fact that babies and young children are whole people. This holistic view of child development means that as an educator one is aware of the context in which the child is living — at both micro- and macrolevels of society — and the influences health, housing, economy, ideology and so on have on children's ability to take up learning opportunities offered.[5,6] The system should not only 'make sense' to the policy-makers and providers, it should 'make sense' to parents and children. After all, just as the Policy and Practice Review Group of the National Children's Bureau[7] stated the importance of parents as primary health carers, so too it is accepted that parents are the primary educators of their children. Bringing together these two elements — health and education — in a child's development and learning the need for support systems for families was perhaps never greater than in the current climate of poverty, parental unemployment, family mobility, divorce and separation.[8-10] How early childhood educators do and can work at the education/health interface will now be considered.

HEALTH AND SAFETY LEGISLATION AND ITS IMPLICATIONS FOR EARLY YEARS TEACHERS

The parents of young children will, first and foremost, wish to be assured that their children are safe when left in the care of others. The Health and Safety Commission's Education Service Advisory Committee produced a booklet,[11] in which they recommended that every school develop and implement its own health and safety policy. The policy should provide staff with details of each person's responsibilities relating to the monitoring of safety standards, regular discussions of accident reporting and investigation, inservice training on new initiatives, and evaluation of policy implementation. The usual rules concerning health and safety representatives apply to nursery and infant establishments. Further, the new inspection system demands such policies.

Early childhood educators must be constantly vigilant about equipment and premises which could be potential hazards to very young children, but the law contains the key phrase 'so far as is reasonably practicable', meaning that staff should have weighed up the seriousness of risk compared with the reasons for leaving the possible hazard in place. For example, should a headteacher decide to rid the nursery of pencils because of the potential risk for a child who may disregard a sensible rule that pencils be used at the table or mat provided? Clearly it is the responsibility of the staff to ensure that the group is run in an orderly manner and that children are given equipment appropriate to their stage of development, and that they are encouraged to use this sensibly.[12] Konner[13] has reported that in other societies very young children are given opportunities to learn the correct use of long and sharp knives. What we decide is inappropriate may tell us more about adult/child ratios in our early years settings, our concept of early childhood and expectations of young children, than about what is endemically dangerous to the young. Perhaps one of the most telling criteria for gauging the importance a society ascribes to its youngest members is the level of awareness of their safety, well-being and freedom. It is not only members of Western European societies who have become more anxious about their young children, their lack of freedom to play outside the home, or to go from one place to another alone, as described in a study of 8-year-olds, 'One false move'.[14] Early years writers in Eastern European countries have expressed the same concern[15] and its far-reaching effects on children's personal and social development.

HEALTH EDUCATION IN EARLY CHILDHOOD

The consultative document 'The health of the nation'[16] contains a clear message that health education, education for a healthy lifestyle, is to be a central strategy in reducing ill-health and promoting behaviour expected to reduce the cost of health services. However, health education is problematic. The main dilemmas centre on the fact that health education is permeated by considerations of values and attitudes.[17] However, health education is a subject that has been recognized as important to primary school teachers. A survey conducted in 1985 indicated that some 87% of primary schools were teaching about health. The figure for nurseries would no doubt equal or surpass this, since the teaching methods used in nurseries include taking up spontaneous, or casual, incidents and elaborating on them in such a way as to effect learning. For example, children will talk about the need for cleanliness when washing their hands, or protection on sharing a story in which people are depicted riding bikes wearing helmets (or not!). This type of coincidental health education continues in nursery and infant classes, and in the nurseries there is still the possibility for time to be spent on planned, thematic work which will include health education elements. For children aged over 5, however, the story during the last few years may be slightly different.

Health education and the National Curriculum

At the time of the inception of the National Curriculum, following the 1988 Education Act, many teachers were concerned because health education had been omitted from the statutory orders. Subsequently, guidelines for five cross-curricular themes were published, and these included health education.[18] Owing to the realization that the total content of the National Curriculum for primary schools in the core (English, mathematics, science with information technology) and basic subjects (history, geography, physical education, art, music) and religious education was 'too big', Sir Ron Dearing was given the task of consulting with selected groups to make the curriculum 'just right'.[19,20]

Although some educationists[21] argue that so much may be discarded that the idea of a national curriculum as an entitlement will be lost, because what remains will become 'too small', there are hopeful messages now emanating from the schools piloting the pruned curriculum. However, the cross-curricular themes were earmarked very early as casualties. Thus, the health education guidelines are not expected to be retained as an entitlement for every child. Furthermore, personal, social and moral education, and physical education, regarded as allied or integral to health education, have been pushed further into the background during the years of initiating the National Curriculum.

Driven as the Government is by an ambition to raise standards in literacy, numeracy and science, in the interests of the economy, a sceptic might argue that there may be more to the narrowed focus of the curriculum than meets the eye, since an exploration of the philosophical bases of health education (see below) highlights its controversial nature.

Different models of health education

Prior to the Leverhulme Health Project in the 1970s,[22] the dominant model of health education was a medical one, predicated upon a portrayal of the human body as a machine which, when ill, could be cured through the wonders of modern science. However, as modern technology proved ineffectual in many illnesses, despite soaring costs, the influence of lifestyles began to be recognized. As a result, health education began to be seen as a vehicle for improving the health of the nation, or at least of future generations, in accordance with this revised medical model, and thus health education as prevention.

A second model of health education sees the role of the education sector as one of developing children's ability to think, to draw their own conclusions — in other words, to make rational choices, given the facts. Thus the Schools Council Project 'Health education 5–13' stated that the main aim of health education should be to help children make considered choices concerning their own health behaviour, rather than merely passing on information.[23] Criticisms of this approach,[17] centre upon the question of 'free choice',[24] especially for those living in poverty, who are often also those least able to articulate and demand what they need. Some visiting Swedish students placed in local schools here in the UK were appalled to observe that staff in schools did not offer advice to parents who sent their children to school with junk food as snacks for breaktime. They felt that those who work with very young children should act as their advocates, upholders of children's right to a healthy diet, because the children themselves are both powerless to challenge and inexperienced in knowing health facts.

The radical model of health education[17] argues that, rather than blaming the victim (i.e. those who become ill, have an unhealthy lifestyle, diet, etc.), there should be an analysis of the root causes of ill-health. Both the Black Report[25] and the Court Report[26] were influential publications which encouraged a re-evaluation of the causes of ill-health, suggesting that policies and programmes to tackle poverty and unemployment would be more appropriate measures than preaching to the powerless.

Tones[17] argues that a self-empowerment model leads on to the concept of each individual having a 'health career', developed through education, which includes teaching about values, attitudes, beliefs and behaviour in such a way that an 'alliance' is forged between social education and life-skills approaches.

Health education programmes which do not pay respect to the fact that parents will have socialized their children about health through both 'teaching' and by modelling behaviours are not only likely to fail, but may place children in conflict situations. For example, the powerful use of certain foods as control mechanisms, or as symbols in gestures expressing love, cannot be underestimated.

This minefield for teachers is further exacerbated by the influence of the media, since advertisements, magazines, film, television, and even computer/video games, often portray food or other behaviour which is inimical to a healthy lifestyle. In fact, researchers report that some teachers continue to be ambivalent about health education, seeing it as the responsibility — or territory — of parents.[27] There are, however, many ways in which, whether they like it or not, schools do contribute to children's health and their health education. The messages conveyed by the 'hidden curriculum' in the status, time-allocation, spending on health education, physical education, personal, social and moral education, and the organization of school mealtimes, together with what is sold in school for snacks, provide children with learning experiences which are imbued with meaning and significance likely to have long-term effects on their health. For example, anyone who has observed the midday mealtime in many of Britain's primary or secondary schools will sympathize with Morrison's distress when gathering research data,[28] and cannot fail to ask themselves the effects such encounters may have upon our children's attitudes towards food and health. In contrast, where they still do provide a midday meal (ie. children may attend full-day), nursery schools and classes can be an oasis of calm and pleasure — powerful examples of non-didactic teaching.

Wetton & Moon[29] argued, even before the implementation of the National Curriculum, that health education has low status and that, further, it is difficult to define. They add that parents and other professionals from the health field are likely to feel they have a right to be involved in the health curriculum offered children. Indeed, medical officers to schools are encouraged, in a publication from their own association,[30] that they should become involved in some of the teaching if they are so inclined, but that they should certainly make sure each school gives health education its proper place in the curriculum, and that the Health Education Council is used as a guide and provider of resources. Reporting on a survey conducted about 10 years ago, Wetton & Moon[29] provide the key areas identified as comprising health education for young children: keeping safe; healthy eating; relationships; use and misuse of drugs; exercise and fitness. Critical concepts and skills for each stage were also identified, as were ways in which learning might be achieved, and ways of negotiating with parents and communities to identify priorities. Additionally, grouping of topics and cross-curricular links were reinforced, and evaluation strategies were provided. The framework was intended to assist in the development of opportunities for interaction between the home, communities and professional groups. In this the ethos of the school would play a crucial part, since self-esteem — of children and their parents — would have a bearing on the success of any such initiatives. After all, the overall aim was to develop the role of the school as a health-promoting community working in partnership with families.

Sensitive issues: sex education in schools

Sex education was at the centre of controversy as a result of news reports and the (then) Secretary of State for Education, John Patten's, intervention. Circular 5/94 sets out the statutory position following changes introduced by the 1993 Education Act. It also gives advice on 'appropriate content and purpose of sex education ... and guidance on the development and implementation of policies on, and programmes of, sex education'.[31]

Governing bodies of schools are required to have a policy statement on sex education. Parents have the right to withdraw their children from sex education classes. However, at the stage under discussion here, teachers are more likely to encounter the occasional enquiry related to reproduction, say, when a pupil's mother is expecting or has just given birth to a baby, or when a pet has a litter. While early years teachers have always attempted to provide sensitive answers to such questions, usually followed-up by a word to parents, they are aware that British parents are not a homogeneous group. They do not all want their children fully informed, although there are increasing numbers who see the sensitive and sensible answering of young children's questions when they arise as the most appropriate way to educate children about sex. To a young child, adult sexuality must be incomprehensible, but that does not mean they are to be kept in total ignorance, nor that they do not have their own sexuality. The 1993 Education Act has made life extremely difficult for all teachers, since during the summer of 1994, the Secretary of State for Education will make an order under this Act to the effect that teaching about AIDS, HIV and anything other than the biological aspects of human sexual behaviour cannot be conducted in a science lesson. Again, looking at what happens in other countries, research by the Goldmans[32] has indicated that the earlier children are informed about sexual activity, in a balanced way, the less likely they are to indulge in early activity with the resultant teenage pregnancies. It seems unfortunate that the Secretary of State imposed his own values on the education system in Circular 5/94,[30] when the working party which developed the guidelines for the cross-curricular theme 'health education',[18] had produced a more appropriate and workable document for the world of today.

Young children's perceptions of health

In a study focusing on 4–8-year-olds, Moon et al[33] explored children's perceptions of what keeps them healthy. Children from 125 primary schools were involved in the survey, in which they were asked by their teachers to keep their ideas 'secret' from their friends and to draw a picture of these ideas. They were then helped by their teachers in labelling what they had drawn — still keeping their 'secrets'. Although around a fifth of the children interpreted the request as 'draw whatever you like', and these responses were discounted, a total of 1225 focused responses were obtained. The largest proportion of these (417) concerned keeping fit and exercising and 346 related to food. Only 23 were concerned with the prevention or cure of illness. Caring for teeth, aspects of hygiene including keeping the home clean, and sleep, were other categories. The researchers concluded that certain educational activities had clearly had an effect on the children's perceptions, especially dental health education.

Organizations offering assistance and support to teachers in developing health education

The Health Education Council, local health promotion units, Relate, and other specialist organizations can often help teachers wishing to educate themselves about a particular issue, or to develop the curriculum for children. TACADE, the Teachers Advisory Council on Alcohol and Drug Education, and the Health Education Council have been especially helpful in training teachers about general health education and about contemporary problems. Although the idea of training early years teachers about drugs and alcohol abuse may seem strange at first, it is often nursery staff who come into regular contact with parents caught up in such difficulties.

HEALTH SURVEILLANCE BY TEACHERS AND OTHER EARLY CHILDHOOD EDUCATORS

Although recent reforms of teacher training courses have led to a serious reduction in the time available for students to study child development, teachers and nursery nurses in particular have put their studies to good use in that they have been able to participate in the identification of children needing special treatment or special education. Early childhood educators will sometimes notice something about a child to which the family have either become accustomed, or have attributed to a different cause. For example, a suspected hearing loss can be quickly checked by an audiologist, after gaining parental agreement. Some parents will have had no way of judging whether their child was simply too intent on an activity to notice their conversation, and most will be relieved that staff care enough to wish to have a check made on a condition which may need attention. While temporary hearing losses as a result of colds are frequent at this age, a more serious condition can have long-term, disadvantageous effects on the child's learning opportunities if left untreated. Sometimes forms of surveillance can be developed as part of the curriculum; for example, regular height and weight checks can be incorporated in many themes and activities in which the children themselves take part.

The importance of the part played by early childhood educators in such surveillance cannot be underestimated. In a sense some are replacing older relatives who would have performed this function for young parents in the past, when the extended family lived in close proximity.[34] Sadly, one area in which their surveillance is most noticeable is that of child protection, children under 5 forming the largest group suffering physical abuse. Further, there is increasing evidence that children in this age group are also subjected to other forms of abuse, including sexual abuse. Perhaps one of the most important functions of nurseries is the way in which they can provide a supportive service to parents who are under severe stress, so acting as a preventive network in a community.[34-37]

Although child protection is an important function of all services for children, and volunteers and professionals are required to work effectively together in children's best interests according to the Children Act 1989, teachers do have some problems concerning referrals. First, school staff are likely to have worked long and hard to establish good and trusting relationships with parents and communities. A referral, especially where the case eventually failed, could break down that trust throughout the local community. Although the intention in the Children Act is for assessment to occur without the need for a court order, parents will still feel they have been betrayed by those they took their children to every day in a spirit of friendship. For the teacher, the dilemma is that a child cannot be allowed to suffer for the sake of home-school relations. Some children will not even disclose to a teacher because they believe the teacher is their parents' friend rather than their own. As a result it is sometimes students, meals supervisors, and others with less obvious power to whom children divulge their secret anxieties. Teachers need far more training, the development of a code of conduct, and greater confidence in the contributions they are qualified to make, in order that they develop positive policies collaboratively with parents and governors, so that everyone involved knows and understands that the school is a community support, but that first and foremost its responsibility is to the children.[35]

In research conducted in Canada,[36] it was discovered that teachers were very lenient in their attitudes towards parental disciplining techniques. They did not always feel they had a right to intervene in or report a case of severe treatment of a child by a parent. Meanwhile, in Sweden, nursery workers are failing in their duty and are sanctioned if they do not report a parent for hitting a child, but the parents would then be offered support to change these behaviours. This example provides us once again with a view of the ways in which different societies adopt different attitudes towards young children and their place in society — do they have rights as people, or are they simply their parents' possessions?

INTERPROFESSIONAL COLLABORATION AND TRAINING

The links between educational and other professionals, including those in the health service, has a long history in the early years sector, but effective liaison between professionals from a health and those from an education background is now required by law under the Children Act 1989. As well as formal links — required medical checks, child abuse case conferences, etc. — many informal links are organized on a local basis,[37] where workers have recognized the need for concerted action, even if there has been little time to discuss shared philosophy.[35]

Health visitors and GPs have a tradition of working closely with their local nurseries, making recommendations for priority entry when families are under particular stress, or children thought to be at risk in various ways. The part played by school nurses and school medical officers cannot be underestimated in both the identification and maintenance of health in individual children and, importantly, in the day-to-day running of a school. Although the frequency and focus of their visits has been reduced in the last 10 years, their expertise and status can be a considerable support to a headteacher and staff seeking remedies to problems in their own schools. Physiotherapists, speech therapists, audiologists have all recognized that there can be gains from meeting the children they are to assess or treat in their school setting rather than in a health centre or clinic. Parents can be advised when they will attend, both staff and parents can support and follow-up their work, and they themselves can see a number of children in one session if necessary. At the same time it must be acknowledged that, like educational psychologists, many health professionals carrying out assessments have realized that the context in which they observe or work with children is very influential. A young child in the play environment of a familiar nursery will be more likely to 'perform' optimally than one in strange surroundings with unfamiliar people using curious equipment.

While arguing for this type of flexible approach on the part of health professionals, it is important to add that teachers do understand the constraints, especially the constraints of too little time and too few resources combined with too much work, which may prevent further development of nursery-based work with parents and children. Further, this is not an appropriate or possible way to handle certain cases. When a child has an accident in the nursery and a parent cannot be contacted, it is usually a teacher who takes the child to the local accident and emergency unit, together with the school's basic health record of that child.

Other contacts between health and education professionals in a health rather than an education setting will include hospital play specialists[38] and teachers, and nurses with a nursery nursing qualification (as well as nursery nursing students) bring educational expertise to obstetric and children's wards of hospitals.

It is not possible here to go into detail about these crossings of boundaries. What is important, however, is an analysis of the issues raised by interprofessional collaboration.[39] When Fitzherbert[40] was writing almost 20 years ago, she stated (p. 20) that what made it

> ... difficult to give a straightforward account of the school health service in early 1976 service is the fact that the service is awaiting recommendations for changes. In 1974 all local authority health services, including school health, were brought under the administrative umbrella of area health authorities, which simply took over the statutory obligations of the school health service and guaranteed to discharge them to their existing standard. Meanwhile a committee was set up under Professor Court to consider how the health services for children, which are now divided between GPs, hospital paediatrics departments and the school and other community health services, could best be organised into a unified service.

Fitzherbert[40] goes on to argue (p. 21) that whatever was to happen to school health services, teachers and their health colleagues should establish relationships 'within which constructive cooperation can flourish'.

One of the problems encountered when Fitzherbert was writing, and which is still recognized today, is the lack of dialogue between health and educational professionals about the children in their care. While this may be the result, in part, of attention to confidentiality and the code of conduct regulating the actions of health professionals — and ethical considerations must be acknowledged by all involved — it can also act as a barrier between professions, and one which may need closer scrutiny as it may not always be in the best interests of the child. As Spencer[39] has pointed out, other professionals may at times collude with physicians to reinforce their own rather superior view of themselves. First, the education sector needs to pay more attention to their need for a code of conduct. This has been reiterated many times by protagonists of a General Teaching Council, fashioned loosely on the model for health professionals. Although a 'shadow' council exists chaired by Professor John Tomlinson, a regular participant in interprofessional bodies and publications (e.g. refs 41,42), there has been continual rejection of this idea by central government.

Secondly, both health and education professionals need to explore their assumptions about the withholding of information on the grounds that it is confidential. Members of a group studying for an advanced diploma in early childhood studies found wide variations in the attitudes of health visitors when they approached them, initially through their managers, with a view to exploring their role in the community. All the students were in senior positions in education, all were very experienced. They were naturally grateful to all five health visitors who agreed to meet them, but what followed for the pairs demonstrated a gulf from one area to another. In the most positive liaison the teacher (the deputy head of a primary school) was invited to accompany the health visitor on her round. It was completely understood that the health visitor might ask the teacher to remain outside, or to leave the home, if this was felt necessary for reasons of confidentiality. In every case the families welcomed the teacher and felt her co-visit was beneficial. This may have been due to the fact that the health visitor had already asked the permission of the parents to bring the teacher with her. This teacher found the shadowing exercise fruitful not only because she now had a greater insight into the tremendous workload of health visitors, the stresses and strains of the job, but also because it gave her insights into aspects of the lives of some of the families of children attending her school, to which she had not previously been party.

At the other extreme, another experienced teacher was told that she would not be permitted to 'shadow' the health visitor contacted, but that she could visit the clinic and questions concerning the role would be answered where possible.

Clearly there is a need for interprofessional training, to enhance mutual understanding of roles, services, expectations. Such understanding has not been helped by the recent far-reaching changes to all the services. These have been difficult enough for a person working in one service to keep up with, let alone someone from another background.

CONCLUSION – THE HEALTH ADVANTAGES OF COMPREHENSIVE EARLY CHILDHOOD SERVICES

Surveys and research concerning the effects of early childhood education provision as a preliminary to primary school for all children[43-45] have emphasized the gains for society in the long term. One facet of these gains, according to American research,[46] is the ultimate saving from the public purse (7 dollars for every dollar spent) through the greater autonomy of the young adults who experienced high-quality preschool education, compared with non-attenders. These savings, which could be seen as a long-term investment in young children, included a reduction in the number of teenage pregnancies; greater involvement in continued education, training and employment, less involvement in crime, drug culture, and so on. In other words, there were direct gains to health costs of the nation as well as, presumably, indirect gains because of the reduced likelihood of living in poverty.

During children's earliest years, perhaps more starkly than in any other period, the lines between health and education workers are blurred — health professionals act as educators and education professionals act as health workers, who care for and about the children with whom they come into contact.

The European Community set out health targets for member states; it also set out a recommendation that they develop a more child-friendly society.[47] This included ensuring adequate daycare and out-of-school facilities, and a safer environment. Governments will have to report on progress in 1995.

Comprehensive surveys of the influence of poverty on children's health[10,24] indicate the important relationship between poverty and child health and, more importantly still, point one in the direction of social policy in its widest sense. It is important, however, to recognize the ways in which our society may not accord young children the priority they merit during this crucial phase in their development.[48]

If we create a society which regards the provision of services, including a midday meal, to very young children and the building of a safe environment as factors which can be left to market forces, we must recognize that there will be long-term costs, because the young have no vote and cannot participate in the market. In such a climate it rests upon those of us in services such as education and health to act as their advocates.

REFERENCES

1 David T. Under five — under-educated ? Buckingham: Open University Press, 1990
2 Moss P (for the European Commission). Childcare and equality of opportunity. London: European Commission, 1988
3 Pugh G. Services for under fives: developing a coordinated approach. London, National Children's Bureau, 1988
4 Pugh G, ed. Contemporary issues in the early years. London: Paul Chapman/NCB, 1992
5 Osborn AF, Milbank JE. The effects of early education: a report from the child health study. Oxford: Clarendon, 1987
6 Bronfenbrenner U. The ecology of child development. Cambridge, MA: Harvard University Press, 1979
7 National Children's Bureau Policy and Practice Review Group. Investing in the future: child health ten years after the Court Report. London: NCB, 1987
8 David T, ed. Working together for young children: multi-professionalism in action. London: Routledge, 1994
9 Bradshaw J. Child poverty and deprivation in the UK. London: NCB, 1990
10 Kumar V. Poverty and inequality in the UK: the effects on children. London: NCB, 1993
11 Health and Safety Committee ESAC, Safety policies in the education sector. London: Health and Safety Committee ESAC, 1985
12 Brierley D. Health and safety in schools. London: Paul Chapman, 1991
13 Konner M. Childhood. London: Little, Brown, 1991
14 Hillman M, Adams J, Whitelegg J. One false move: a study of children's independent mobility. London: Policy Studies Institute, 1990
15 OMEP/UNESCO. The universal and the national in preschool education. Paris: UNESCO/OMEP, 1994
16 Department of Health. The health of the nation. London: HMSO, 1991
17 Tones K. Health promotion, affective education and the personal and social development of young people. In: David K, Williams T, eds. Health education in schools. London: Harper Education, 1987
18 National Curriculum Council. Health education. York: National Curriculum Council, 1990
19 Dearing R. Review of the National Curriculum: interim report. London: NCC/SEAC, 1993
20 Dearing R. Review of the National Curriculum: final report. London: SCAA, 1994
21 Campbell J, Neill SStJ. Stress for little gain. Child Educ 1994; 71(6): 5
22 Leverhulme Project Team. Report on the Leverhulme Project on Health Education, 1978 (cited in ref. 17)
23 Schools Council. Schools Council Health Education Project (SCHEP). London: Nelson, 1977
24 Blackburn C. Poverty and health: working with families. Buckingham: Open University Press, 1991
25 Townsend P, Davidson N. The Black Report: inequalities in health. Harmondsworth: Penguin, 1982
26 Committee on Child Health Services. Fit for the future. Report of the Court Committee Cmnd. 6684. London: HMSO, 1976
27 Reid D, Massey DE. Can school health education be more effective? Health Educ J 1986; 45(1): 7–14
28 Morrison M. Eating in school: mincing words about educational experience. Paper presented at the CEDAR International Conference, Warwick University, April 1994
29 Whetton N, Moon A. Health education in primary schools. In: David K, Williams T, eds. Health education in schools. London: Harper Educational, 1987
30 Medical Officers of Schools Association. Handbook of school health. Stoke-on-Trent: Trentham Books, 1992
31 DFE (Department for Education). Education Act 1993: sex education in schools. Circular 5/94. London: DFE, 1994
32 Goldman R, Goldman J. Show me yours: what children think about sex. Harmondsworth: Penguin, 1988
33 Moon A, Whetton N, Williams DT. Perceptions of young children concerning their

health. In: Kelly PJ, Lewis JL, eds. Education and health. London: Pergamon Press, 1987

34 Ferri E, Saunders A. Parents, professionals and pre-school centres. London: NCB/Barnados, 1991

35 David T. Early years teachers and child protection. Buckingham: Open University Press, 1993

36 Tite R. How teachers define and respond to child abuse: the distinction between theoretical and reportable cases. Child Abuse Neglect 1993; 17(5): 591–604

37 Whalley M. Learning to be strong: setting up neighbourhood service for under-fives and their families. London: Hodder and Stoughton, 1994

38 Barnes P, Rathburn B. Your heart operation. Burnley: Children's Heart Federation, 1994

39 Spencer N. Multi-professionalism and the Children Act: a paediatrician's view. In: David T, ed. Protecting children from abuse. Stoke-on-Trent: Trentham Books, 1994: p. 39–46

40 Fitzherbert K. Child care services and the teacher. London: Temple Smith, 1977

41 Tomlinson J. Attitudes to children: are children valued? Early Years 1991; 11(2): 39–42

42 Working Group for the Gulbenkian Foundation. One scandal too many: the case for comprehensive protection for children in all settings. London: Calouste Gulbenkian Foundation, 1993

43 National Commission on Education. Learning to succeed. London: National Commission on Education, 1994

44 Ball C. Start right: the importance of early learning. London: RSA

45 Osborn AF, Milbank JE. The effects of early education: a report from the Child Health. Oxford: Clarendon Press, 1987

46 Schweinhart LJ, Weikart DP. A summary of 'Significant benefits: the Perry Preschool Study through age 27'. London: High/Scope UK

47 Cohen B. A programme for Europe. Child Educ 1993; 70(2): 11

48 Currer C. Understanding the mother's point of view. In: Wyke S, Hewison J, eds. Child health matters. Milton Keynes: Open University Press, 1991

9. Teachers' awareness and role in childhood chronic illness

M.J. Bannon

TEACHERS AND THE 'IN LOCO PARENTIS' ROLE

'Teachers ban first aid for peanuts allergy boy' ran the alarming headline in the quality broadsheet newspaper (Sunday Telegraph, 3 July 1994). The article described the plight of a boy with allergies who was forced to leave his playgroup because teaching staff were apparently unwilling to accept responsibility for the administration of intramuscular adrenaline in the event of him experiencing an episode of anaphylaxis. Similar events have been documented in both local and national press with regard to teachers' reluctance to give rectal diazepam to children who have epileptic fits. Situations such as these, in which conflict is evident between parents and teachers regarding administration of medicines to children in schools, are not uncommon and they frequently result in deadlock. This is a sad state of affairs as each of the protagonists involved would state that they were acting in the best interests of the child concerned.

Parents' views

Parents would quite reasonably expect that their children should receive the same level of care and supervision while they are at school as they would at home and this might include protection from preventable physical harm as well as an acceptable level of discipline. Some parents would remind teachers that they have traditionally held an 'in loco parentis' role with regard to the supervision of children who are in their care. Furthermore, parents of children who have chronic disorders such as asthma, epilepsy and diabetes are aware that these illnesses have the potential of impairing learning through lost school days and that the effects of many illnesses such as asthma persist throughout school hours. Some parents would require that their children receive medical care on a 24-hour basis to include the time they are at school and would argue that administration of medicines could be considered part of an extended 'in loco parent's role. Parents, in addition, have high expectations and can invoke the support of an ever-increasing number of parent support groups who are willing to undertake an advocacy role on the part of individual children.

125

Teachers' views

Teachers, on the other hand, clearly have rights too. No other professional group would be expected to undertake activities which could have potentially serious outcomes without either adequate training or support from both employers and professional trade unions. Teachers would put forward the view that administration of medicines is not generally perceived to be part of their role and in any case few teachers will have had specific training on the subject of medicial illness in childhood. As one teacher said: 'We are teachers not doctors'. The term 'in loco parents' is at best vague and is prone to misinterpretation. The term itself is old and recent legal opinion states that the term is misleading in its characterization of the source and nature of the teacher's authority and fails to take into account recent developments.[1]

Children's rights

In all of this conflict and debate it must not be forgotten that the paramount issue is that children also have rights and it is a joint responsibility of agencies and professionals that the special needs of individual children are met. The United Nations Convention on the Rights of the Child recognizes the inherent right of disabled children as well as children with illness to access appropriate medical are, and also emphasizes the right of children to the highest level of health possible.[2] The Children Act 1989 states clearly that agencies should work in partnership in order to reduce the adverse effects of childhood illness and disability.[3] A key issue, therefore, is the precise role that teachers may usefully undertake in the care of children with illness. The philosophy of both of the previously mentioned documents would indicate that care for children with illness should be continuous, to include time spent in school.

School children spend a considerable part of their waking day in school and during this time they are supervised by teachers. Chronic disease in childhood is relatively common. One in five children has some form of asthma and Table 9.1 illustrates the mor ecommon disorders that might be encountered among a population of older school children.

It is likely therefore that most schoolteachers in mainstream schools will encounter some of these childhood disorders on a regular basis. In addition to common chronic disorders, the trend following the implementation of the

Table 9.1 Common disorders encountered among 10–12-year-olds (Rutter, Isle of Wight Study)

Disorder	Prevalence per 1000
Asthma	23.2
Eczema	10.4
Epilepsy	6.4
Diabetes mellitus	1.2

1981 Education Act has been for an increasing number of children with less common but more complex physical and neurodevelopmental disability to be taught in mainstream schools.

A first step in resolving some of the issues relating to teachers' role in childhood illness would be to determine a number of issues:

- Teachers' current levels of knowledge and awareness of the subject in general.
- Their attitudes towards the school medical service and health-related issues in general.
- Their perceptions of the most appropriate role they could undertake with regard to illness in school children.

A number of isolated studies have been undertaken in this area and the results of this research will now be collated, hopefully in a positive effort to find the best way forward that will protect the interests, rights and responsibilities of all concerned parties.

THE SCHOOL MEDICAL SERVICE AND TEACHERS' VIEWS OF IT

A casual lay observer would state that the solution to some of the problems previously described was obvious: surely the school medical service with its dedicated team of doctors, nurses and administrative staff was ideally placed to resolve any difficulties that might arise with regard to the administration of medicines in school and other child health related issues? The problem is that the school medical service, since its inception in the early years of this century, has been preventive rather than therapeutic in its clinical focus.[4] The need for a preventative school health service whose function was to reduce the effects of disease and disability among school children was recognized and the 4-minute routine medical examination represented the hallmark of the school medical service. The function of the routine inspection was not only the early detection of unsuspected defects but also the provision of information which would guide education authorities with respect to overall development of children while they were at school.[5] Hence the need for proper communication between teachers and the school health service was acknowledged. Communication was later emphasized when the concept of educational medicine was endorsed by both the Court[6] and Warnock[7] Reports. 'Educational medicine' embraces the study and practice of child health in relation to the process of learning. The key elements of educational medicine activity would include two-way communication between teachers, doctors and nurses whereby medical staff are alerted to the unmet medical needs of children and the attention of teachers is directed towards children with unmet educational needs resulting from known or newly discovered handicap or chronic disease. It is indeed sad that, as the research will show, the desired levels of communication have in many cases never been established.

A second limitation of the school medical team of doctors and nurses is that it is not a resident service nor has it ever been. Medicals are undertaken on a rotary basis between different schools and both doctors and nurses will be designated for several schools.

A small but illuminating survey was undertaken by Fitzherbert in 1982.[8] Interviews were conducted among 35 junior teachers to determine their general knowledge of health services available for school children and teachers were also asked about coverage of health-related subjects during their training. The results demonstrated that teachers have a limited appreciation of the school health service in terms of its structure, activities and functions. Information about the medical support services available for children in school did not feature prominently in their training. Communication between teachers and medical staff was in general poor and parents were the main source of information about individual children's medical problems. The teachers surveyed were critical of their own ignorance but deplored poor communication between themselves, parents and doctors. Similar findings regarding teachers' source of information were found in a survey of spina-bifida children in mainstream school in another study.[9]

Lack of information and poor communication are two identified problems which seem to have persisted over the years. Fox et al[10] in South Belfast attempted to identify the way schools perceive the school health service and identify teachers' concerns as well as their suggestions for improvements. They found that teachers had a poor level of knowledge concerning the school health service and that they would positively welcome more information. The teachers also complained of poor communication between medical and teaching staff.

Another survey conducted in Macclesfield yielded similar findings.[11] Teachers were given the opportunity to state their views regarding the school medical entrant examination as well as their views of other health-related topics. The majority of teachers viewed the school medical examination favourably. Table 9.2 shows the sources of information concerning individual children with parents representing the most common source.

The majority of responding teachers favoured meetings as means of disseminating information, but over half wanted written information as well.

Table 9.2 Sources of information for teachers regarding childhood illness in Macclesfield (Jones & Gordon[11])

Source	Percentage of respondents
Parents	32.3
School doctor	22.8
Nursery nurse	11.4
School nurse	8.2
Educational psychologist	8.2
Others	17.1

Most teachers in Macclesfield expressed a wish for general medical information on medical, behavioural and emotional disorders. Unfortunately, the school nurse had a low profile in the views of the teachers sampled. The authors conclude by recommending that printed information should be available for teachers on what the school health service has to offer and on diseases such as asthma, diabetes, epilepsy and general health. A useful suggestion was that teachers' perceptions of the school health service might be an appropriate subject for audit.

TEACHERS' KNOWLEDGE OF SPECIFIC COMMON CHRONIC CHILDHOOD DISORDERS

A limited number of studies have been conducted by health professionals which have aimed to assess teacher knowledge and perceptions of specific childhood illnesses. There are thus in existence a number of papers which assess teacher knowledge of diabetes, asthma and epilepsy. While these papers have been published from different sources using different teachers as their subject material, the studies are remarkably similar in the following characteristics:

- They attempt to assess teachers' detailed medical knowledge of various childhood illnesses.
- They try to identify sources of information for teachers on various aspects of childhood illness including levels of previous training.
- They ask teachers to state whether or not they are interested in learning further about the illness being surveyed and also regarding their preferred method of teaching.
- Analysis of the results of these surveys also attempts to relate teachers' personal experience and years of teaching experience with the level of knowledge they have regarding the individual illness.

Asthma

A study in 1988 was conducted by Reynolds et al in which 224 school teachers in South Sefton Health Authority were asked to complete a questionnaire which determined their knowledge of childhood asthma.[12] The results showed that 82% of responding teachers underestimated the incidence of asthma, and 36% were unaware that exercise could trigger an attack; 44% were unaware that medication was needed as a treatment for an acute attack, and (a minority) 22% of teachers considered that they should be involved in the administration of treatment at school. Almost all of the teachers surveyed would have liked to be better informed regarding childhood asthma. It was also found that older and more experienced teachers were more likely to give appropriate advice to asthmatic children regarding exercise. An alarming finding was that overall teachers would cope badly if a child had an acute asthmatic attack in school, or on a school trip. Nearly 50% of responding teachers were unaware that asthma could be fatal. A conclusion was that teachers should be better informed about asthma and be better equipped to deal with an acute attack with less doubt and anxiety.

In 1990, a survey was conducted by Bevis & Taylor among 98 primary school teachers in London which also demonstrated limited understanding of asthma and its management.[13] Few teachers had received any teaching or training about asthma and they considered the arrangements for giving antiasthmatic drugs in schools as unsatisfactory. They also considered that administration of drugs caused unnecessary disruption to the child's school life. A positive attitude on behalf of the teachers was revealed in that they correctly believed that asthmatic children are of similar intelligence to others and all of the teachers thought that asthmatic children should be educated in normal schools. In that particular study there was no significant difference in responses between experienced and less experienced teachers, although in this study 3 years' teaching experience was taken as the cut-off limit. It was found that school policy on medicines varies considerably and teachers were often unaware of their own school's policy. Less than half of the teachers would permit children to keep their inhalers with them because of concern about overdose and other complications. The authors recommended that all primary school teachers should receive teaching about asthma during their teacher training with regular in-service training for those working in schools.

Diabetes

Bradbury & Smith conducted a questionnaire survey in Merseyside in order to determine teachers' knowledge of childhood diabetes.[14] They found that just 25% of the teachers surveyed had an adequate understanding of the medical aspects of diabetes and that diabetic pupils and parents, rather than the school medical service, were the most common source of information regarding children with diabetes. Teachers who had greater than 20 years of teaching experience were less likely to be anxious when presented with a diabetic child than more junior colleagues. Those teachers who had personal knowledge of other diabetics scored better in the general knowledge questionnaire. Disappointingly, leaflets were not fully effective in informing school teachers. An encouraging finding was that teachers themselves appreciated the need for more knowledge regarding diabetes and that they felt literature of a brief nature would be most appropriate, followed by in-service courses or talks and visits by health professionals. They particularly asked for information on the recognition and treatment of diabetic emergencies. In their conclusions the authors state that, in order for children with diabetes to achieve their educational potential, it is not unreasonable for teachers to have some knowledge of the more practical aspects of diabetes. The authors concluded that the poor level of understanding of childhood diabetes reflected failings in communication within the local medical service.

Some years later a similar study was conducted in Birmingham, which attempted to investigate teachers' knowledge and sources of information regarding diabetes.[15] The study also tried to identify the benefits of peripatetic diabetes nurse specialists, with regard to improving the awareness of teaching staff. Results were rather similar to those of Bradbury & Smith, in that only one-third were found to have an overall adequate knowledge of diabetes. Teachers' total knowledge scores were found to be positively related to the number of sources of information about diabetes they were exposed to, and those teachers who knew at least one other person with diabetes scored higher knowledge scores. Interestingly enough, the mean knowledge score of female teachers was higher than that of their male colleagues. In the Birmingham study no relationship was found between teachers' total knowledge scores and number of years spent teaching. In only a minority of cases were teachers given information by the school nurse or doctor, and most of their information came from other school staff and special case information sheet provided by the diabetes nurse specialist. The vast majority of teachers indicated that they would like to know more about diabetes and its management in relation to the child at school.

Epilepsy

In a similar fashion, information and attitudes held by teachers regarding childhood epilepsy has also been studied. One of the best known is that published by Holdsworth & Whitmore[16] in 1974. In the course of their enquiries into the welfare of 85 children known to have epilepsy who were attending normal schools, they asked the head teachers concerned regarding their attitudes towards children with epilepsy as well as the amount of information they possessed for individual children. The researchers found that teachers were unaware of 36% of epileptic children in their schools. In 18 instances teachers first became aware of epilepsy when the child had a fit in school. In 53 cases teachers were told of children's epilepsy, the source of information being as follows: parents (25 cases), previous school (6), school health service (22), child's seizure in school (18), other sources (7). With regard to appropriate action for teachers to take in the event of a child having a seizure in school, teachers had apparently learned what to do from previous experience, general knowledge or from first aid training. In general, teachers were willing to accept children with epilepsy but stated that they would feel more at ease if they had received instruction about what to do in the event of a major seizure. The teachers welcomed more information about children with epilepsy and the need for better communication between teachers and doctors was clearly demonstrated.

It is a source of disappointment to note that little seems to have changed with regard to levels of communication between the school medical service and teachers concerning the dissemination of information concerning school children who have epilepsy. A more recent study based in North Staffordshire and which was undertaken among 142 school teachers revealed that respondents did not feel confident when teaching children with epilepsy and only a minority considered their knowledge of the subject to be adequate.[17] The majority of teachers did not consider that children with epilepsy were more likely to have problems with learning and their views regarding correct restrictions to be placed on the activities of epileptic children were overall appropriate. Despite a lack of previous training on epilepsy, teachers appeared to know what to do in the event of a child suddenly having a fit in school and their general knowledge regarding childhood epilepsy was adequate. The main finding from the Staffordshire study was that relating to teachers' confidence. Only 5% felt very confident when supervising a child with epilepsy and those teachers who had either previously witnessed a fit or who had a friend or relative who had epilepsy were more likely to be confident. Communication between parents, teachers and the school medical service was poor. Nearly half of the respondents were made aware of a child's epilepsy when he/she had a fit in the classroom and regrettably in only 14% had prior discussions taken place between doctors and teachers.

It would appear that childhood epilepsy presents particular difficulties for teachers. Despite media coverage and efforts by the British Epilepsy Association, epilepsy is still a misunderstood and sometimes feared condition. It unfortunately possesses a stigma and parents may be reluctant to share information with anyone other than their own paediatrician and GP. Teachers in all of the surveys who have witnessed fits have found the experience frightening. A new dimension has been added by the common practice by paediatricians of prescribing rectal diazepam for the immediate treatment of individual seizures, especially where status epilepticus is likely to occur. While there is no doubt that, in certain circumstances rectal diazepam can be an extremely effective form of treatment, it is unreasonable perhaps to expect all teachers to assume responsibility for this form of treatment.

OTHER ASPECTS OF CHILD HEALTH

Surveys of teachers' knowledge of issues relating to all aspects of child health have now become more common and include broader topics, such as those discussed below.

Child abuse

Although child abuse might not be strictly considered to be an illness, it is an important child health and welfare issue where teachers may play an important role. Abrahams study from the USA revealed that, in that country, teachers received a minimal amount of education on identifying, reporting and intervening in suspected cases of child abuse and most teachers considered the level of education to be insufficient.[18] While the majority of American teachers were willing to report in principle cases of suspected abuse or neglect, 65% stated that a significant obstacle was a lack of sufficient knowledge of child abuse in general as well as familiarity with local guidelines. This survey highlighted deficiencies in the US system of training and provision of support for teachers. This could well reflect a problem peculiar to the USA, but could have implications for teachers in this country and represents an area for future research.

Accidents

Accidents represent the most significant source of mortality and morbidity in the age group of children who are attending school. The subject area of accident prevention is an important one and has been highlighted in the 'Health of the nation' document.[19] Although schools have been traditionally viewed as providing a safe environment for children, it has already been demonstrated that accidents frequently happen to children while they are at school.[20] A survey undertaken by Carter et al in North Staffordshire among a sample of 278 head teachers showed that the majority of respondents agreed that accident prevention was a suitable subject to be taught in schools but only a minority felt that they had enough background information on the subject.[21] The teachers particularly requested first-aid instruction. Almost all respondents maintained an accident log-book at school but there was considerable variation with regard to both accident recording and reporting. Older teachers were more likely to promote safety literature and larger schools were more likely to give safety leaflets compared to smaller ones.

Health promoting schools

Most developed countries have endorsed the philosophy of the World Health Organization's global strategy 'Health for all by the year 2000'. The goals of the strategy are to be achieved through the application of the principles of primary health care with particular focus on health promotion and illness prevention. The notion of a health promoting school has been developed by some countries as a result of the 'health for all' strategy. A 'health promoting school' has been defined as one which has 'policies, practices, and programmes that promote and support the health of students and other members of the school community'.[22] In health promoting schools, the role of teachers is extended to include a contribution to the proper management of a full spectrum of common childhood disorders. It is also recognized that teachers are well placed to promote children's health in general.

Australian schools have been recently identified as ideal venues in which to promote children's health.[23] Research conducted among 234 teachers in New South Wales attempted to ascertain whether teachers understood their potential as primary health carers. The questionnaire survey also examined teachers' perceptions of their current level of knowledge related to children's health needs and common childhood disorders and identified means whereby teachers could increase their knowledge. The results were remarkably similar to those obtained in the previously described UK studies. General knowledge relating to the school health service was limited and interestingly enough the level of this knowledge was not related to age or experience of responding teachers. Teachers appeared to have a poor understanding of their role in health promotion. Compared to UK studies, school nurses were more available to Australian teachers, had a higher profile and were much appreciated; 91.6% of teachers in the representative sample requested future instruction in health-related matters. Seminars in school settings were much favoured as well as short courses.

SUMMARY OF FINDINGS FROM ABOVE STUDIES

Detailed meta-analysis of the above studies is not possible because of differences in research methodology, but overall common themes are evident which can be summarized and represent a useful starting point in improving the overall situation.

Teachers' knowledge of child health issues

In general, knowledge of chronic childhood illness by teachers is not adequate. The exception to this generalization in the papers surveyed would be the survey on attitudes to childhood epilepsy conducted in North Staffordshire.[17] Teachers in that study appeared to have an adequate overall knowledge of childhood epilepsy, which might have resulted from a chance finding but it must be remembered that the teachers sampled in that study were relatively mature in years of teaching experience. The studies have in addition revealed a lack of awareness and understanding of the school health service in general in terms of its purpose and what it has to offer.

Previous training on child health issues

It is not surprising that teacher knowledge and awareness on the issues discussed is so poor as few teachers have had specific instruction either during their training or in service when qualified. This is no criticism of the teachers involved and one wonders how well school medical doctors would fare on questionnaire surveys regarding their knowledge of the educational system! Despite lack of training as well as lack of communication from the medical profession some teachers do have surprisingly good knowledge of childhood illnesses which unfortunately appears to have been acquired as a result of personal experience. This situation appears not to have improved despite the profusion of excellent educational material produced by such voluntary organizations as the British Epilepsy Association and others. Excellent awareness and training packages are available on asthma, diabetes and epilepsy. Printed material alone from various sources would therefore appear to be relatively ineffective in increasing both confidence and awareness among teachers.

Teachers' attitudes towards children with chronic illness

The outstanding feature of all these surveys is the positive attitude of the teachers studied. They seem to recognize that children with chronic illness have a right to education in the mainstream setting and that individual illnesses such as diabetes or epilepsy should not prevent children from attaining their potential. They would also appear to be critical of their own lack of knowledge and almost unanimously want more instruction on chronic childhood illness. The exact method of such instruction varies according to the particular group of teachers studied and includes such options as in-service training, seminars, meetings with medical staff and written information.

Communication between the school health service and teachers

Communication between teachers and the medical profession would appear to be inadequate in most instances and non-existent in others. This is still the case despite stated changes in focus of the school health service to concentrate its efforts on the needs of the relatively few children with special needs.[24] It is now also recognized that parents hold the prime responsibility for provision of care for their children and hence would be expected to communicate with teachers. However, it seems unacceptable that parents still represent the main source of information for teachers regarding children's illness. Communication difficulties therefore exist at two levels: between teachers and school health staff, and between hospital paediatricians and school doctors. This difficulty persists despite the institution of integrated child health services in some districts and the appointment of consultant community paediatricians.

The way forward

In the determination of a positive way forward, several potential areas of difficulty are evident. More than one survey has urged that teachers should receive a minimum of instruction on childhood illness while they are being trained. Increasing teacher awareness of the relevant issues previously discussed would represent an ideal situation which teachers themselves would welcome. At present, this does not seem to be a feasible option in the UK as considerable changes are evident in the way in which teachers are trained with less time spent in theory and more in practical teaching in the classroom.[25] In addition to this, the school medical service in many districts is being generally run down. The school health service represents a logical source of support for teachers but it is under threat due to financial constraints. Teachers' trade unions have in general been cautious in the advice they have given to teachers regarding whether or not individual teachers should take responsibility for the administration of medicines to children. Finally, there is always the ever present issue of confidentiality. While active communication between all interested parties is to be encouraged, there are often occasions when parents do not wish information to be shared beyond that of their GP or paediatric consultant. This has been particularly the case with regard to childhood epilepsy. Areas of potential difficulty concerning communication between the school health service and teachers are summarized in Table 9.3.

A POSSIBLE WAY FORWARD

General considerations

An appropriate and proper role must be both defined and accepted for teachers with regard to the health of school children under their supervision. Teachers represent a caring and responsible profession who could offer more to the health of children apart from their goodwill. It is unfortunate that so much attention is focused upon the difficult issues of administration of such drugs as rectal diazepam and intramuscular adrenaline when there are broader and perhaps even more important health-related matters to be considered. As a matter of some urgency, a nationally agreed role must be established for teachers in this area and this should be a collaborative initiative between all interested parties: education, health, teachers' unions as well as parental support groups and the voluntary sector. The agenda for discussion for such a forum would be diverse, interesting and perhaps controversial but would conceivably include some of the following topics.

1. Teachers if properly empowered could become useful members of the school health surveillance team by virtue of the fact that they supervise large numbers of children for considerable periods of time. Most paediatricians will be familiar with situations whereby astute teachers have alerted the school doctor to previously unknown cases of asthma, temporal lobe epilepsy and other important medical conditions.

2. They could also ensure that children with such chronic illnesses as asthma and diabetes can lead school lives which are as normal as possible. For example, if teachers have an appreciation of the relevance of dietary factors in diabetes and the effects of exercise on children with asthma, then they are more likely to understand the difficulties and constant challenges that children with these illnesses encounter.

Table 9.3 Areas of potential difficulty

- Changes in teacher training
- Uncertain future of the school health service
- Attitudes of teacher professional trade unions
- Parental views on confidentiality

3. Teachers are well placed to fulfil a definite role in health promotion with regard to issues such as those outlined in 'Health of the nation' as well as the 'health promoting schools' initiatives. The National Curriculum has addressed this in part, but more emphasis could be placed on their role regarding child accident prevention, sexual health, exercise and smoking.

4. A commonsense and non-contentious approach is needed with regard to the administration of medicines to school children by teachers. Situations where conflict between parents and teachers reaches the press represent a failure of trust and communication which in the long term will only ensure that all parties involved become entrenched. It is unlikely that the best interests of anyone involved will be served. The term 'in loco parentis', therefore, is unhelpful and perhaps either needs redefinition or should be avoided altogether.

Specific issues

The question arises as to who should take the lead in resolving the present difficulties, bearing in mind that the problems are complex and long established. National agreement is needed at central level between the agencies involved, but it is obvious that at present we are still some distance away from such negotiation. My argument therefore is that responsibility for resolution falls by default to the local school health service who could achieve much on a patch basis. It should be feasible for most such departments to address some of the following strategies.

Increasing teachers' awareness

A key objective should be to ensure that teaching staff have a proper understanding of the local school health service, how it works and what is has to offer. Locally relevant written information would be of benefit and could be used in association with presentations and meetings. Teachers' views of the local school medical service should be regularly canvassed in the form of a joint audit project and their observations should be taken into consideration.

Understanding of specific chronic illness by teachers can be achieved in a number of ways. Regular training events on the more common illnesses to include asthma, diabetes and epilepsy can easily form part of a school-based training event which could be held in localities and updated on an annual basis. In my experience, such voluntary organizations as the British Epilepsy Association, British Diabetic Association and Asthma Foundation can offer much in the way of experienced speakers who not only are knowledgeable on the medical aspects of the illnesses concerned but can also provide advice on specific and relevant educational problems. Such voluntary organizations will also provide written and audiovisual material to consolidate these training sessions. Some additional written guidance for teachers will also be needed. Most local educational authorities will have available to them some written guidelines on medical illness of childhood. An informal audit of such material locally has revealed them to be deficient in many ways and out of date. It should be a responsibility of the community paediatrician or school health doctor who acts as adviser to the education authority to ensure that such documents are not only relevant and up to date but that they are widely available and circulated among school staff. Such written advice should also describe the local school medical service.

Inevitably, children with significant but less common disorders than those described above will be placed in mainstream schools. An ad hoc approach would be successful and feasible whereby written information regarding the child's illness would be made available for school staff including definition of appropriate action which would be required by teachers in specific circumstances.

In addition to the above measures, local schools of education could be approached as some training at postgraduate level might also be possible.

Communication

Increased levels of communication will only be possible if all of the involved parties are aware of each other's role and appreciate the positive contribution that everyone can achieve in the care of individual children. There is much support for the concept of a patch-based school health team which by extension should include teachers. The 'community paediatric team' represents a parallel that has been described elsewhere.[26] Effective teamwork ensures both adequate communication in addition to mutual respect. One aspect of successful teamwork is that of regular meetings between members whose purpose includes exchanging ideas and keeping each other informed. Hospital paediatricians when treating childhood illness should be aware of possible implications for schools. With this in mind, some districts have found it useful for school medical officers to attend specialist diabetic, asthma and oncology clinics, and have also appointed specialist school liaison nurses. The Personal Child Health Record is a powerful communication tool which could facilitate communication between doctors of all grades, parents and teachers, and could perhaps play an important role in this regard.

Support for teachers

Doctors have been accused of delegating much of the responsibility for the surveillance and management of school children to teachers.[8] Nowhere is this more evident when the subject of administration of drugs to children becomes relevant. While it is not unreasonable to expect teachers to have a better knowledge of childhood illness and to be aware of the implications of illness in a school setting, it is somewhat unrealistic to expect them to automatically assume responsibility for the administration of drugs to children. A reasonable approach would assume the following:

- No teacher should be forced to assume a medical responsibility that they do not feel comfortable with.
- If a teacher is willing in the interest of an individual child to assume such responsibility, then appropriate training should be provided as well as explicit written guidance.
- The teacher concerned should have the full support of the employing education authority in the event of a mishap. Some education authorities have insisted that parents sign an agreement that indemnifies the teacher and have also written an indemnity policy in general. However, the legal status of indemnity has yet to be tested.
- Occasionally the situation will arise where a child might need immediate medical treatment in school and teachers do not feel they can undertake a medical role. Cases such as these represent a challenge, and support for that child in school must be provided in some other way, e.g. classroom assistant.

In addition to the above local solutions, lobbying at a more central and national level is needed. This should be part of the advocacy role of community paediatricians. It is encouraging to find that the functions and activities of the school medical service is receiving the attention it deserves as a result of the recent British Paediatric Association discussion document.[24] Hopefully the whole issue of teachers' role in medical illness will then be addressed. The school medical service has left teachers relatively unsupported for far too long and has relied too much on teachers' goodwill. In the meantime the school health service at a local level must do what it can in order to ensure that children receive the standards of care they are entitled to while they are at school.

KEY POINTS FOR CLINICAL PRACTICE (Table 9.4)

Table 9.4 Local solutions to the problems

Problem/challenge	Possible solutions
Ill-defined teacher role	• Nationally agreed role for teachers in health surveillance, enabling of children with illness and health promotion • Abandon the term 'in loco parentis'
Increase teacher awareness	• In-service training days • Written guidance and information on the school health service • Meetings
Improve communication	• Establish a patch-based school health team • Regular meetings • Use of personal child health records
Support for teachers	• Commonsense approach to the administration of drugs in school

REFERENCES

1 Crook H. In loco parentis: time for a reappraisal? Fam Law 1989; November: 447–449
2 United Nations. Convention on the rights of the child. New York: UN Department of Public Information, 1991: Annex II, Article 24
3 The Children Act. London: HMSO, 1989
4 Whitmore K. The past, present and future of the health services for children in school. In: Macfarlane JA, ed. Progress in child health. Edinburgh: Churchill Livingstone, 1984: vol 1
5 Board of Education. Memorandum on medical inspection of children in public elementary schools. London: HMSO, 1907
6 Court SDM. Fit for the future: report of the Committee on Child Health Services. London: HMSO, 1976
7 Warnock HM. Special educational needs: report of the Committee of Enquiry into Education of Handicapped Children and Young People. London: HMSO, 1978
8 Fitzherbert K. Communication with teachers in the health surveillance of school children. Matern Child Health 1982; 7: 100–103
9 Halliwell B. Spina bifida children in normal schools. Child Care Health Dev 1977; 3: 389–405
10 Fox TK, Rankin MG, Salmon S, Stewart MS. How school teachers perceive the school health service. Public Health 1991; 105: 399–403
11 Jones C, Gordon N. The school entry medical examination. What do teachers think of it? Child Care Health Dev 1992; 18: 173–183
12 Reynolds MA, Aylward P, Heaf DP. How much do school teachers know about asthma? Pediatr Rev Commun 1988; 2: 173–180
13 Bevis M, Taylor B. What do school teachers know about asthma? Arch Dis Child 1990; 65: 622–625
14 Bradbury AJ, Smith CS. An assessment of the diabetic knowledge of school teachers. Arch Dis Child 1983; 58: 692–696
15 Warnes J. Diabetes in school: a study of teachers' knowledge and information sources. Pract Diabetes 1988; 5: 210–215
16 Holdsworth L, Whitmore K. A study of children with epilepsy attending ordinary schools. II: Information and attitudes held by their teachers. Dev Med Child Neurol 1974; 16: 759–765
17 Bannon MJ, Wildig C, Jones PW. Teachers' perceptions of epilepsy. Arch Dis Child 1992; 67: 1467–1471
18 Abrahams N, Casey K, Daro D. Teachers' knowledge, attitudes and beliefs about child abuse and its prevention. Child Abuse Neglect 1992; 16: 229–238
19 The health of the nation. London: HMSO, 1992
20 Dagano A, Cabrini E, Anelli M et al. Accidents in the school environment in Milan, a 5 year survey. Eur J Epidemiol 1987; 3: 196–201
21 Carter YH, Bannon MJ, Jones PW. The role of the teacher in child accident prevention. J Public Health Med 1992; 16: 23–28
22 Smith C, Nutbeam D, Roberts C, Macdonald G. The health promoting school: progress and future challenges in Welsh secondary school. Health Promot Int 1992; 7: 171–181
23 Thyer SE. Health promoting schools: primary school teachers' perceptions of their need for information related to child health issues [unpublished report]. Faculty of Health, University of Western Sydney, 1993
24 Polnay L Consultation report of the joint working party on health services for school age children. London: British Paediatric Association, 1993
25 Department of Education and Science. Expansion of school based teacher training. London: DES, Press release May 1992, 158, 92
26 Polnay L. The community paediatric team — an approach to child health services in a deprived inner city area. In: Macfarlane JA, ed. Progress in child health. London: Churchill Livingstone, 1984: vol 1

10. Delivering comprehensive child care services in general practice

J. James

Child care services in general practice are developing and improving rapidly. The changing nature of general practice over the last decade — the emphasis on providing preventive services, the development of the team approach, closer working relations with secondary services, and increasing specialist training for general practitioners (GPs) — has resulted in a service that is ideally placed to adapt to the needs of children in the 1990s. The majority of child surveillance now takes place in general practice, a result of close teamwork between paediatricians and the primary care team. This, however, is only a beginning. By developing this partnership, and by considering the true health needs of children, there is an opportunity to provide truly comprehensive health care services for children. The challenge is exciting.

In this paper I shall consider first the true health needs of children and propose a philosophy of care. One in four children in the UK now live in poverty, and are considerably disadvantaged. Their health needs merit special discussion. After reviewing the services currently provided for children in general practice, I will suggest additional services that we should be offering to children today. In the final section I will propose a possible way forward in order that these aims may be achieved. These relate principally to improved access to primary care services, reallocation of workloads within the primary care team, comprehensive data collection, to setting standards of good practice, to targeting resources to those most in need, to targeted interventions and for research. Without major changes in social policy, children's health will remain compromised by deprivation, and advocacy on their behalf is an essential component of achieving true health for children.

If GPs and community paediatricians can work in partnership, combining their skills of knowledge of the family and the community, of all aspects of child health, of epidemiology, of research, of teaching and communication, and of advocacy, children's health services will develop considerably.

THE HEALTH NEEDS OF CHILDREN

In 1981 the World Health Organization's (WHO) 'Health for all children by the year 2000' declaration[1] heralded the concept of 'true health' for children.

WHO considered not simply the physical, but complete 'mental and social well-being' of children. The British Paediatric Association has declared the aim of paediatric services to 'enable as many children as possible to reach adulthood with their potential uncompromised by illness, environmental hazard or unhealthy lifestyle'. The 1989 UN Convention on the Rights of the Child[2] demands that children 'enjoy the highest attainable standards of health. . . without discrimination of any kind'. The UK Government, in their first report to the UN Committee in 1994,[3] confidently claimed that the UK's policy, law and practice met the provisions of the convention; the British Association for Community Child Health (BACCH) in a discussion document on behalf of the British Paediatric Association find many provisions sadly lacking.[4] Many children in the developed world do not enjoy good health.

Until these timely declarations were made, 'health' was equated with 'lack of disease'. Thus a child who was free of physical illness, who was immunized against specific and potentially life-threatening diseases, and who was free of disability could be considered 'healthy'. Consequently, a well-developed 'reactive' health service could be considered to provide comprehensive care. This myopic view took no account of the influences on health of poverty and deprivation, of family disharmony, of psychological stress and the need for programmes of health promotion.

Thus the onus on health professionals to broaden their horizons is considerable. There is a need to promote a healthy lifestyle for families, to empower parents, and to work towards healthier and safer communities. The discrepancy in health outcomes between children from different social backgrounds in the UK should concern all those working with children.

From this, however, it is possible to develop a philosophy of child care. Children are our future, and have the right to develop to their full potential. Health targets for children could be based on the concept of equity: that is, to enable all children to achieve the health outcomes of children from wealthier backgrounds. This could be achieved by targeted interventions and by advocacy for sociopolitical change.

Children's health needs are primarily met by their parents, and much can be achieved by those in primary care by offering a family orientated service, based on partnership and empowerment. An understanding of the additional pressures of hardship and stress will enable medical services to achieve these health aims for children.

THE ADVERSE EFFECTS OF POVERTY ON CHILD HEALTH

Increasing numbers of children living in poverty

Child poverty is an increasing problem in the UK. In 1979 Townsend[5] introduced the concept of relative poverty: 'the lack of resources to obtain the types of diet, participate in the activities and have the living conditions and amenities which are customary in the society to which they belong'. Families living in 'relative poverty' have a disposable income of less than half the national average disposable income. This has the advantage of clear definition, and allows for international comparisons. In 1990, 24% of all children living in the UK were living in relative poverty, compared with 18% in 1980 — an increase of 26%. This compares with an increase of just 13.9% in the European Community. It is for this reason that the effects of poverty on health merit discussion.

Children and poverty

Poverty affects not just morbidity but mortality.[6] Judge & Benzeval[7] have demonstrated a three-fold increase in mortality in children aged between 1 and 14 years between social classes I and II and those children whose parents are unemployed. Their figures suggest that 200 children may die each year due to the cumulative effect of this social disadvantage. The variation in morbidity data suggests the same social class divide. The prevalence of accidents, failure to thrive, chronic respiratory disease, non-accidental injury and hospital admission is similarly increased.

Interest has recently focused on the long-term sequelae of ill-health — particularly in the field of nutrition. Barker[8] has shown an increased prevalence of ischaemic heart disease, cerebrovascular accident, hypertension and non-insulin-dependent diabetes in adults who had been underweight at birth or underweight at 12 months of age. Both factors are associated with low socioeconomic status. Iron deficiency anaemia is a common condition,[9] with a prevalence of up to 25% in 1-year-olds from deprived backgrounds. It is associated with developmental delay[10] and, although the delay appears reversible with treatment with iron, longer term follow-up suggests the delay may persist. These children will be permanently disadvantaged.

Poverty and family life

The effects of deprivation and the breakdown of family life have considerable influence on the health and emotional well-being of the carers of children too. Depression, low self-esteem, adverse health behaviours (smoking, alcohol and drug abuse) and domestic violence are all negative influences on the ability to care for the child. Environmental influences — poor housing, lack of play areas, inadequate child care provision, pollution — are further pressures on the carer. This is reflected by the increase in behavioural disorder seen in children today.

Furthermore, primary care provision in deprived areas is often poor. General practice services are often limited, and the primary health care teams may be poorly resourced, working from substandard premises. Perhaps most important of all, those living in deprivation are poor users of health services, often not understanding how to access resources, even though their needs may be great. Members of ethnic minority groups are at particular risk.

All these considerations must be taken into account when planning more comprehensive services in general practice.

GENERAL PRACTICE SERVICES FOR CHILDREN TODAY

Services for children

- Reactive service
- Gatekeeping
- Immunizations
- Child surveillance for under-fives
- Parent-held records

Positive developments in general practice

- More GPs trained in hospital paediatrics
- Improved postgraduate education in paediatrics
- Improved liaison with community paediatricians
- GPs learning teamwork — working with health visitors, etc.
- Computerized records

Changes and pressures in general practice

- Fundholding — GPs as purchasers
- Health promotion targets
- Less out-of-hours work (deputizing services used)
- Resources not targeted to deprived areas

Child care services in primary care

Child care services offered by GPs are developing rapidly. Traditionally, GPs offered comprehensive, though purely reactive, services for children and their carers; until recently, surveillance, immunizations and health promotion have been provided by community child services. GPs have a role of 'gatekeeper' — determining which children receive secondary care — services that until now have been separated from primary care. GP training schemes — no doctor can become a principal in general practice without completing the scheme satisfactorily — require 3 years of hospital training before 12 months' training in general practice; most doctors spend 6 months in a paediatric unit. As a result, most practices will have a partner who has had paediatric training. An increasing number of GP trainees have a postgraduate paediatric qualification (DCH or MRCPaed).

The majority of practices now offer comprehensive immunization programmes, as well as child surveillance for preschool children. This has enabled practices to develop well-baby clinics suited to the needs of families; uptake of services is high (uptake of immunizations nationally exceeds 90%). Community paediatricians have been able to develop closer links with GPs as a result of offering training courses in child surveillance; many now offer outreach secondary services based in health centres.

Postgraduate education in paediatrics

There is now greater emphasis on postgraduate education for GPs: GPs are expected to complete 10 half days of approved postgraduate education every year. In 1991, 60% of 620 GPs working in Avon replied to a questionnaire sent out by the Institute of Child Health at the University of Bristol: 60% had spent at least 6 months in hospital paediatrics, and 75% would be 'very interested' in attending paediatric postgraduate meetings; 10% expressed an interest in forming a paediatric research group. As a result of the survey, paediatric study days have been introduced in addition to child surveillance courses and are well attended. A general practice paediatric research group has been established; ten GPs meet quarterly with paediatricians, and a number of research projects are under way.

Computers in general practice

At present, 70% of general practices have installed computer systems in their practices. Initially introduced to improve practice management, practices record basic information on each patient registered (downloads are available from Family Health Service Authorities (FHSAs)). Most practices record immunization data; computerized prescribing is commonplace; many practices are compiling morbidity data. A computer screen is a familiar sight in many consulting rooms, as GPs realize their benefits. All systems are capable of storing very large amounts of morbidity and sociological data. There is great potential for data collection.

GPs are realizing the importance and benefits of teamwork. In the field of child care, GPs, health visitors and practice nurses are working together, sharing casework, recognising each other's specialist skills. As a result, child surveillance and immunizations are carried out in a team setting with benefits for staff and children.

Pressures in general practice

There are, however, a number of pressures in general practice. Practices have needed to develop their management skills, and much time is spent dealing with administration. GPs derive nearly half of their income from items of service. Immunizations are one example. Each immunization attracts a payment; there is an additional payment if the practice attains a nationally determined uptake (currently 90%). Practices serving deprived areas often find these targets difficult to attain; in spite of increased workload, no additional resources are targeted to these needy practices. Furthermore, there is disillusionment with many of the 'health of the nation' targets, which are not universally seen as being appropriate, but which must be attained to gain the financial rewards they attract. the development of fundholding (most practices will be fundholding by 1996) has meant practices are handling large budgets for the first time. Negotiation with providers is very time consuming.

Finally, GPs are increasingly disillusioned with out-of-hours work. Many practices rely on deputizing services (available in many large towns and cities) with the result that there is less continuity of services for children. It is likely that the majority of out-of-hours work will be offered from designated health centres, with less emphasis on home visiting. This may impact on accident and emergency departments in general and paediatric hospitals.

CHILD SERVICES THAT GENERAL PRACTICE COULD BE OFFERING TODAY

Adoption of a new philosophy of child care

- Equity for all children
- Child care in the context of the family setting
- Recognizing that the parent is the principal carer for the child
- A pro-active service for all age ranges
- Developing services based on the needs of the local community

Essential services

- Standardized management of common diseases
- Appropriate referrals to secondary services — involvement in ambulatory paediatrics
- Structured programmes of health promotion — nutrition, healthy behaviours
- Psychological support and advice for children and their carers
- Development of community care plans for children with disability
- Support for children on child protection register
- Coordination of community-based care for long-item or life-threatening illnesses
- Adolescent services — support and advice
- Specialized services appropriate to practice population needs
- Advocacy for appropriate resources based on practice population needs

Guidelines for the management of common conditions

Up to 70% of GPs' consultations with children are concerned with common infectious diseases, for which no clear management guidelines exist. Parents will often experience inconsistent advice and treatments from different GPs, who may often work in the same practice. They will be confused as to the best management and many will choose to consult with a particular GP who offers treatment that accords with their own view. This is a particular problem in dealing with treatment of infections of the upper respiratory tract where there is considerable debate as to the role of antimicrobials. This may also be true when arranging secondary referral; in the management of secretory otitis media, for example, where there is little consensus by paediatricians as to optimum management, GPs themselves may determine management by referring to a particular surgeon with a known preference.

Health promotion guidelines and priorities

Few would argue that health promotion should form an important part of GPs' workload, yet lack of guidelines, a dearth of health promotional materials and time constraints result in little advice being offered. There is a need to prioritize key areas for health promotion — nutrition, healthy behaviours, accident prevention, for example — and of ensuring that consistent advice is given by all members of the primary health care team.

Managing behavioural disorders in children

Behavioural disorder in children is an increasing problem in general practice. GPs should be able to offer support and advice to children and their parents and carers; they should be able to identify those children who will require specialist services.

Children with disability

One in ten children in the community has a disability. All should have a care plan; GPs should be involved in their planning and execution. Children with life-threatening, or chronic, illnesses have special needs; where possible these children should remain at home, and their needs should be met in the community. Again, the needs of those children who are on the Child Protection Register should be provided for in general practice.

Adolescent health

Adolescents and teenagers are poorly served by general practice. Structured services, particularly focusing on healthy behaviours, should form an essential component of general practice. GPs should be able to identify problems in child health that relate to their own practices, and be able to advocate on families' behalf for appropriate resources.

Addressing the needs of families

Finally, GPs should develop services that are appropriate to the needs of the families with whom they work. This will require working more closely with families, and close liaison with other agencies in the community.

THE WAY FORWARD

Philosophy

- Resources targeted to communities most in need
- Interventions based on local needs
- Deprived children have the right to the health outcomes of children from wealthier backgrounds

1. Improved access to primary care
2. Reallocation of workload in primary care
   - Greater role for health visitors and practice nurses
   - Ambulatory paediatrics
   - Nurse practitioners
   - Health promotion workers based in health centres
3. Establishing standards of good practice
   - Greater use of parent-held records
   - Protocols for management of common illnesses
   - Provision of extra services
     Adolescent health
     Responding to local need
     Health promotion
4. Data collection
   - Morbidity data
   - Practice profiling
   - Feedback, audit
5. Interventions
   - Targeted to local needs
   - Based on empowerment
6. Education and support for primary care teams
   - Closer working with secondary services
7. Research
8. Establishing desirable health outcomes for children
   - Measurable
   - Achievable

Improved access to primary care services

Child health services in the community will not be improved unless all children have equal access to primary care. There is a need for improved facilities in deprived areas, both in terms of premises as well as allocation of staff. There must be recognition that many families are poor users of health care systems — often using emergency services inappropriately, yet under-using preventive services. The development of ambulatory paediatrics is exciting, and may provide useful opportunities for teamwork between paediatricians and GPs. There may be a role for GPs working alongside paediatricians in these units.

General practices must provide clear guidance about the services that are available for children; they must ensure that they are available and accessible at all times. Much depends on teamwork within the primary care team and recognition that receptionists (usually the first point of contact with the health centre) are important members of the team.

Establishing standards of good practice

There is a need to establish standards of good practice. First, there is a need to develop consistency in the management of common illnesses. This should lead to the development of common protocols, to be used by both doctors and nurses. Health visitors and practice nurses are well placed to advise on the management of these illnesses; it is likely that many parents and carers will then be able to manage common viral infections at home, releasing additional consultation time. In addition, by working more closely with paediatricians, it should be possible to establish guidelines on appropriate secondary referral algorithms. GPs will become more confident in dealing with problems, which will lead to fewer inappropriate referrals. It could be anticipated that practices could develop their own information packs on the management of common problems that could be used by all child carers; input from local community paediatricians would be invaluable.

By developing shared protocols, there is a great opportunity for developing the roles of the practice nurse and of health visitors. Nurses would require little extra training in order to develop their diagnostic and therapeutic skills; there is scope for nurse-run surgeries running in parallel with GP surgeries. Practices should be canvassing actively for nurse practitioners, as well as employing health promotion experts who would be based in health centres.

There is a need to develop additional services. Adolescents and teenagers have important, unmet health needs. They must have access to carefully structured, confidential, sensitive services, focused on their sexuality, health behaviour and taking responsibility for their own health. If these services are to be introduced successfully, there is a need for educational materials and for training for health professionals themselves. Behavioural disorder in children is an increasing problem, and requires specialist skills. General practice is ideally placed to meet these needs, but specialist training will be required. The whole area of health promotion is neglected in general practice; there is a need to appoint key members of the primary health care team to focus on health promotion — accident prevention and nutritional advice being two key areas.

Data collection

Perhaps the most exciting possibility in general practice is the facility to collect data using computers. All practices are likely to be fully computerized within the next 3 years. Uptake of a number of services is already audited (e.g. immunizations); it will be possible to record morbidity data, sociological data, as well as data of specific interest. From a local perspective, this will provide information about services offered, as well as providing profiles of the practice population. This could be used to determine resource allocation, and determine special needs. Centrally collated, the data are already used for feedback (immunization uptake, for example). If there was consensus on important morbidity data, there is an opportunity to develop a comprehensive database which could prove an invaluable research tool in order to learn more about the natural history of disease. This is an exciting opportunity for community paediatricians, epidemiologists and GPs.

Targeted interventions

There is a need for targeted interventions. By identifying specific needs, at-risk populations, and by working closely with families, small interventions have been shown to be very effective. Local knowledge of families and of the community is essential. Again, community paediatricians are ideally placed to offer support and advice. Screening for iron deficiency anaemia has been successfully introduced into deprived communities,[9] and a number of nutritional interventions introduced.

Postgraduate education

There is an opportunity for the expansion of postgraduate paediatric education in primary care. As well as providing study days in postgraduate education, there is an opportunity for team-based education in health centres. Distance learning materials, including computer-aided learning packages, are now available. Paediatricians should strive to visit health centres regularly, and meet up with doctors and nurses. Specific topics may be addressed, but practical skills may also be taught. Community paediatricians now offer outreach clinics in selected health centres, and these have proved popular with staff and patients. Informal meetings encourage the exchange of information and experience, allowing GPs to influence the secondary services offered.

Establishing research priorities and appropriate health outcomes for children

The opportunity for research has already been mentioned. The Department of Health Central Research and Development committee on research and development priorities for the National Health Services in relation to mother and child health will report shortly. Meanwhile it is essential that measurable, important health outcomes for children are determined. These could provide the basis for setting targets for children's health. Until such time, the discrepancy in morbidity and mortality between children of different social backgrounds should provide an impetus for improving child care. There must be recognition that much of the discrepancy will require sociopolitical solutions and that the introduction of such changes will require considerable advocacy. GPs, paediatricians and epidemiologists must recognize that advocacy is a necessary component of child care.

Conclusion

Child care in general practice is undergoing considerable change. By working closely with GPs, paediatricians have the opportunity to develop and influence the future of the delivery of care for children into the next century.

KEY POINTS FOR CLINICAL PRACTICE

Child care services in primary care today

- One in four children in the UK live in relative poverty. This is associated with increased morbidity and mortality in childhood, and the effects impact into adult life.
- Health resources are not targeted to these children.
- GPs are taking greater responsibility for child services in primary care. Many have paediatric training, and are involved in child surveillance. They are learning to work as part of a team, both with colleagues in primary care, with community paediatricians and other agencies. Computerization in general practice has resulted in improved data collection and audit.

Opportunities for child care services in primary care

- Development of a philosophy of child care based on the principal of equity — the right of every child to the health outcomes of children from wealthier backgrounds.
- Closer teamwork between primary care and community paediatricians. The development of agreed common aims, services based on local needs, local targets and targeted interventions. Development of common protocols for disease management.
- Data collection using practice computers. Research opportunities based on morbidity and sociological data, as well as the evaluation of targeted interventions. Data may be used to determine additional resources, and provide a tool for advocacy for children.
- Development of postgraduate education — greater integration between hospital and community, and opportunities for research.

ACKNOWLEDGEMENT

The author is grateful to Dr Tom Bailward for his helpful comments during the preparation of this chapter.

REFERENCES

1 World Heath Organization. Global strategy for health for all by the year 2000. Geneva: WHO, 1981
2 Convention on the Rights of the Child adopted by the general assembly of the UN on 20 November 1989. Command paper 1976: treaty series: 1992: number 44
3 The UK's first report to the UN Committee on the Rights of the Child. London: HMSO, 1994
4 BACCH working group on UN Convention on the Rights of the Child: Implementing the UN Convention on the rights of the child within the National Health Service: a Practitioner's guide 1995. Joint Publication: Children's Rights Development Unit, British Paediatric Association and Royal College of Nursing (in press).
5 Townsend P. Poverty in the UK. Harmondsworth: Penguin, 1979
6 Spencer NJ. Child poverty and deprivation in the UK. Arch Dis Child 1991; 66: 1255–1257
7 Judge K, Benzeval M. Health inequalities: new concerns about the children of single mothers. Br Med J 1993; 306: 677–680
8 Barker DJP. The foetal and infant origins of adults' disease. Br Med J 1990; 301: 111
9 James J, Laing G. Iron deficiency anaemia. Curr Paediatr 1994; 4: 33–37
10 Idjradinata P, Pollitt E. Reversal of developmental delays in iron deficient infants treated with iron. Lancet 1993; 341: 1–4

11. Services for children in residential care

C. de Cates, U. Trend, S. Buck, Y. Ng, L. Polnay

Throughout history, children who live outside their natural family have been disadvantaged in the past, often poorly cared for in the present and with poor prospects for the future. They are a vulnerable group of children who lack advocates and who frequently fail to receive the best that health, social services and education can provide. They are among the most needy and deprived people in our society.

Dr Stephen Wolkind, Consultant Psychiatrist at the Maudsley Hospital, London, has emphasized the difficulties in caring and planning for these children, and the lack of research into their medical and educational needs.[1]

Large numbers of children are involved. As at 31st March 1992, 55 000 children were being looked after by local authorities, with 7600 placed in residential homes. Preliminary figures for 1993 suggest that there will be a reduction in both numbers.

CHARACTERISTICS OF 'LOOKED AFTER' CHILDREN

Deprivation is a common factor among children who need to be looked after.[2,3] Prior to being looked after by the local authority, young people may have been subjected to physical, sexual and emotional abuse and neglect (Tables 11.1, 11.2).

As adults, young people who have been looked after have a generally, although not universally, poor outcome:[4,5]

1. A combination of uncorrected health problems, poor educational achievements and maladjustment means that they are more likely to be unemployed. Even if employed, they are more likely to be in temporary or casual jobs.[6,7]

2. 37% of all young offenders are amongst those in care or who have recently left.

3. Women who have been in care are more likely to be in their teens and unmarried at first pregnancy, score higher on the Malaise Inventory (a screening device for detecting neurotic ill-health), have a significantly

Table 11.1 Common characteristics of children needing to be 'looked after'

Only a quarter lived with both parents
Almost three-quarters of their families were on income support
Only one in five lived in owner occupied housing
Over one half lived in 'poor' neighbourhoods
Overcrowding (linked with large families)
Parents were of different racial origins
Disrupted family relationships
Parental ill-health, especially mothers
More likely to have been born to young mothers
More likely to have been premature at birth
Less likely to have attended infant welfare clinics
Tended to be lighter and shorter than other children
Found to have a higher prevalence of developmental, behavioural and health difficulties
Poorer school attendance and educational attainment

Table 11.2 Routes into residential care (1985 SSI inspection of community homes)

Neglect
Physical, emotional and sexual abuse
Commission of delinquent acts, offending
Being beyond parental care
Family breakdown
Violence within the family
Repeated rejection
Numerous changes of carer before admission to LA care
Truanting from school
Solvent misuse, misuse of drugs, or alcohol
Self mutilation or suicidal episodes

---

higher rate of psychiatric disorder during the early years of parenthood, and interact less with their very young babies.[8]

Their own children are, in turn, more likely to have behavioural problems in school.[9]

Young people looked after in residential care are even more vulnerable than other young people looked after in general. The majority are adolescents, 70% over 13 and 35% over 16 years. Reasons for residential care rather than placement with a foster family include:

1. being unable to cope with the intimacy or demands of a family care setting
2. failed foster placements
3. being in trouble with the law, for example: being on remand, committed for trial, detained in care

They are likely, therefore, to have a higher prevalence of problems generally, and in particular even more emotional and behavioural problems than the whole group of children looked after.[10–13]

The majority (80%) are in community homes maintained or assisted by the local authority. The remainder are in voluntary homes, hostels, private homes, maintained or independent boarding schools, NHS hospitals, mental nursing homes and penal institutions.

On the whole, young people in homes have not been in care as long as the child care population overall — 40% have been looked after for less than 1 year, but there is a high turnover. They may have had several different placements over a short space of time — 40% of young people leaving care at 16 or over have had 5 or more placements in care. Because of this lack of continuity, and the deprived background from which they came, they have often received poor health care for a long period before and after entering residential care.[14]

Bamford and Wolkind's (1988) report on the physical and mental health of children in care concluded that those who had been in care were gravely disadvantaged as a group, with higher risks of psychiatric ill health and social deviance than any other easily identified group in our society. However, we know very little about the physical and psychological health of children in care, and we need good data collection. They felt that the emphasis of research should be on the preventive aspects of child care.

They identified problems which may contribute to the poor health care of these children (Table 11.3).

Young people in residential care are even more likely to have had a series of carers than children in foster care, and even once settled in a residential home may not have one person who knows them intimately and knows their past history. They are likely to have missed routine surveillance and immunizations. Chronic conditions may have been unrecognized or under-treated. Their higher risk of psychiatric ill health, low self-esteem and depression, and high rate of risk-taking behaviour, self harm, overdoses and intoxication, does not lead to targeting of mental health services. They are more likely to experience unwanted pregnancies and sexually transmitted disease.

A further problem to which attention has recently been drawn, particularly in the media, and which has serious implications for the health of young

Table 11.3 Problems contributing to the poor health care of 'looked after' children (Bamford & Wolkind 1988)

The lack of any one person intimately familiar with the child's history or alert to symptoms which ordinary parents would notice.
Medical examinations on admission or during placement were undervalued or over looked, and may fail to provide relevant information.
Medical histories of children in care were usually 'grossly inadequate' and seldom include an interview with the parents.
The value and importance of growth charts in assessing the child's overall well-being was not sufficiently recognized, although pointed out by the Maria Colwell report in 1973.
Little use has been made so far of the large amount of data potentially available from the analysis of medical records.

people in residential care, is the increasing number of younger adolescents who are absconding and taking to the streets.

It appears that childhood prostitution is increasing.

GIRLS ABUSED ON STREETS LABELLED PROSTITUTES
Schoolgirls who are forced to sell their bodies on city streets to survive are being punished and labelled prostitutes rather than protected as victims of sexual abuse, according to the Children's Society.

(Press release August 1993)

More young people over 16 are turning to prostitution as a means to survive, and through contact with peers, younger children, as young as 11 or 12, may become involved. The lack of education and formal qualifications may subsequently prevent a young person leaving prostitution (Table 11.4).

Young people who have been abused and rejected by their families and end up in residential homes are more at risk. They may find it very attractive to

Table 11.4 Survey on child prostitution

One of us [SB] conducted a small survey in 1993 to assess the extent of prostitution amongst girls and boys in one Midlands town.

Police: It is not an offence for boys to solicit, so there are no statistics for boys. Before 1992 there were about 5 girls under 16 cautioned each year by the police. In 1992 there were 14, and in 1993 there were 23. When cautioned, young girls have a police record. The anti-vice squad has limited resources, and we were told that juvenile prostitution was not a priority.

Community homes: 6 girls and 4 boys from one community home were working the streets. 13 of the 22 girls arrested in 1993 were in the care of the local authority (police statistics). Supervision and control is increasingly difficult in community homes. There are resource limitations within social services and physical restraint has been abolished. Pimps target children in community homes, and young people already working the streets coax or coerce others to join them. An additional concern is young people sexually abusing other young people. 50% of victims of sexual abuse who were accommodated in community homes were either abused for the first time in the community home, or re-abused there (personal communication). Research suggests that some young prostitutes have been victims of more serious sexual abuse than the general population. Our survey suggests that young people who have been abused and rejected by their families are at greater risk of becoming prostitutes.

Genitourinary clinic: The consultant and health advisor who specialize in work with young people were seeing a few under age girls in prostitution, but had not seen any boys.

Education Welfare: One officer in an inner city area knew of 6 girls and one boy who were not attending school and were involved in prostitution.

Community child health: Of 30 doctors who were surveyed, 5 were aware of 9 girls and 4 boys. Another 6 boys were suspected of being involved in prostitution.

The media: Journalist Nick Davies (*Mail on Sunday*, 21.11.94) referred to 3 boys and 6 girls aged from 10 to 15. Mr Davies seemed well informed, and situations described were known to local professionals.

White children far outnumbered black children in this small survey. None were noted to have physical disabilities but some did have learning difficulties. Assumptions are made that the girls are heterosexual and the boys are homosexual.

Most of the published research is from North America, and most of it is based on work with older prostitutes.

Table 11.5   Summary of the health problems of young people in community homes

Likely to have missed routine surveillance and immunization
Lack of detection and follow up of chronic medical conditions
Poor school attendance, therefore less access to health promotion and personal/social education (PSE) at school
Emotional and behavioural problems: the original trauma from abuse, neglect and deprivation may be compounded by their experience in care
High prevalence of risk-taking behaviour
Smoking: only 1 out of 12 young people surveyed in one community home in Nottingham was a non-smoker
Substance abuse, drugs, alcohol, solvents
Higher prevalence of unwanted pregnancy, poor antenatal care, and preparation for parenthood
Sexually transmitted infections, including Hepatitis B, HIV, and cervical cancer
Those on the streets or involved with prostitution may be at greater risk of many of these, and at great risk of physical injury from violence, and accidental injury

have a little power from money, and to feel wanted, but be in no position to appreciate the risks (Table 11.5).

SERVICES FOR 'LOOKED AFTER' CHILDREN

Children looked after by the local authority are, in general, a very special group of young people who need a specific service to target their needs.

More than 10 years ago, it was recognized that there were problems with the care offered to this very needy group of young people. The British Paediatric Association (BPA) gave evidence to the House of Commons Social Services Committee which, under the chairmanship of Renee Short, looked into these problems. It concluded that the health care of these children was not of the quality it should be. They suggested that medical problems were commonly given too little attention, citing lack of continuity and lack of liaison between Social Service departments and Health services as contributing to this. They highlighted problems with the medical examination of children on reception into care, and the purposes for which this is carried out. They also emphasized the difference between the first medical, on or very shortly after coming into care, which is meant to detect acute illness, infection and abuse, and the later, more comprehensive assessment of general health and development, in order to plan for the future needs of the child.

The committee made specific recommendations about how the health care of children looked after could be improved (Tables 11.6, 11.7).

However, despite the fact that these problems were highlighted in the recommendations of the Short Report, in practice little subsequently changed in the way the medical care of 'looked after' children was viewed by social services and carried out by health professionals.

In 1988, Madeleine Simms, working at the Institute for Social Studies in Medical Care,[15] looked at the procedures for medical care of 'looked after' children and concluded the following:

Table 11.6 Recommendations of the Short Report 1985

Children should be medically examined on the day of reception into care
Parents should have a right to be present at the examination
Parents not accessible at the time of the examination should meet the examining doctor as soon as possible thereafter
Examination at the time of reception should generally be by the child's family doctor,
but in some circumstances examination by a clinical medical officer or consultant paediatrician may be more appropriate
Social service departments should have designated clinical medical officers and consultant paediatricians
Children who are not certain to return to their parents in 6 months should have a full assessment of health and development, akin to those undertaken before placement
for adoption, and using similar forms, and done by doctors with special experience of child care and development
Examiners should be particularly concerned with growth and development, which should be carefully recorded
A suitable form of examination is required
Forms similar to those devised by the British Agencies for Adoption and Fostering (BAAF) should be required by regulation

1. There is no uniformity in the health surveillance of these children
2. The desirability of a National Code of Medical Practice for children in care
3. The appointment of a designated doctor to co-ordinate the health care
4. The difficulties of overlap in the duties of the general practitioner, clinical medical officer, and consultant paediatrician in the care of these children and the apparent lack of integration, and lack of definition of the qualifications and training required
5. The importance of an allocated social worker in supervising any medical referral that is made, ensuring that specialists are seen and any recommendations made are actually carried out.

Children Act 1989 (Table 11.8)

More recently, the Children Act 1989 has produced innovative changes in the provision of services for children in need, and has profound and far reaching implications for children in care. It emphasizes the necessity to identify and meet the needs of the individual child, ensuring that a child's welfare includes all aspects of a child's health and development. In the case of children in residential care, it has highlighted the legacy of deficient health care which children bring with them to the children's home. In order to compensate for this, residential care staff need to be very aware of the young people's health needs, and play an active role in ensuring that all aspects of their health and well-being are promoted.

There is an emphasis on a high quality, planned, pro-active approach to health care using normal NHS services, not simply restricted to treatment of illnesses and accidents, but including health promotion and education on a wide range of health related topics.

Table 11.7   BAAF (British Agencies for Adoption and Fostering)

The British Agencies for Adoption and Fostering Medical Group (BAAF) is committed to the principle of applying equally high medical standards in all areas of child care work, and has devised forms and practice guidelines which meet the needs of children looked after by the local authority as well as those placed for adoption. The forms are designed to meet statutory requirements, and to provide a basis for the integrated collection of medical information on these children, focusing on the needs both of children and their parents and carers. Practice notes are available, offering guidance to medical advisers and social workers regarding the use of the forms currently available.

The forms include the following:

Form R	The preliminary report on children to be looked after, provides a simple history and examination form, to constitute a baseline of information on all children looked after, and is intended for use on, or as soon as possible after, coming into care, unless the child has been medically examined in the last 3 months.
	BAAF recommends that all young people who remain looked after for longer than 4-weeks, who have repeated admissions, or who may have suffered neglect or injury, should have full medical examination and developmental assessment, using one of the following forms as appropriate:
Form C	Medical report and developmental assessment of child under five years.
Annex to C	Profile of behavioural and emotional well being of child, aged one to 5 years.
Form D	Medical report and functional assessment of child aged 5 to 10 years.
Annex to D	Profile of behavioural and emotional well being of child aged 5 to 10 years.
Form YP	Medical report and functional assessment of young person of 11 years and over.

The following have been developed for information for carers and young people themselves:
MH   Medical history card
My Health Passport.   Health record for children and young people.

The Children Act, however, has retained the statutory requirement for regular medical examinations.

Since the Children Act, and despite the recommendations made in the reports cited above, there is still no consensus view about what health assessment of young people looked after should include.[16] The aim of the initial medical assessment of 'looked after' children and of the regular annual medicals remains unclear.

Medical services for 'looked after' children

There is a lack of guidelines about who should carry out the initial health assessment, what training or experience they require, and what areas of health should be covered. Some medical examinations are carried out by GPs, others by community paediatricians. There is a wide variation between different areas in the amount of involvement of community paediatric services and

Table 11.8 Children Act 1989. Summary of the guidelines relating to 'looked after' children, and in particular those in residential care

---

Responsible authorities should act as good parents in relation to the health of children looked after or accommodated by them

The responsible authority's plan should include health care arrangements, which should be kept under review, including any specifically recommended and necessary immunization and any necessary medical and dental attention

Responsible authorities are required by regulation 7 to arrange for a medical examination and written health assessment of a child. The aim of this requirement is to provide a comprehensive health profile of the child and provide a basis for monitoring the child's development whilst he is being looked after or accommodated

Regulation 6 requires medical examination and written health assessment during placement at least once every 6 months up to the child's second birthday and annually thereafter

Health care implies a positive approach to the child's health and should be taken to include general surveillance and care for health and developmental progress as well as treatment for illness and accidents The health care of all children looked after should be provided in the context of the child health surveillance programmes in the area which are designed to provide child health surveillance and promote the physical, social and emotional health and development of all children

In the case of children with disabilities and those with special needs, consideration must be given to continuity of specialist care

An informed and sensitive approach is especially necessary for 'looked after' children, since they will often have suffered early disadvantage and may be at risk because they have not received continuity of care

Children in homes are particularly vulnerable as they frequently have not received continuity of health care because they have been subject to a sequence of moves often within a fairly short time scale The health of children in homes is likely to be even more in need of attention than that of other children looked after by local authorities

In order that deficiencies in past medical care may be remedied, care staff need to adopt a very vigilant attitude towards the health of children in homes Staff should play an active role in promoting all aspects of a child's health. Health care should include education about alcohol and other substance abuse, sexual matters, and HIV/AIDS and should not be restricted to treatment of illnesses and accidents

Responsible authorities and district health authorities should make arrangements for professional advice to be available to interpret health reports and information, assist in preparing and reviewing arrangements for health care and assist in decisions relating to the child's care One way of providing for this would be to agree that a designated doctor should undertake this work

Regulation 5 requires health authorities to be notified of each placement. Responsible authorities and health authorities should together aim to develop effective arrangements for the communication of information relating to a child's health to all health professionals who are involved with the child

---

child and adolescent psychiatry. Some areas use BAAF forms as recommended by the Short Report, others use locally devised forms which vary in the amount and type of information requested.

The initial examination is:

1. Often refused by the child
2. Undertaken in many cases without any detailed history
3. Perceived as a routine chore

A survey was carried out by one of us (CdeC, MSc thesis, 1991) of the medical reports carried out by general practitioners for one local authority. One hundred names of children who had recently come into care were identified by a senior social worker. For these 100 children, only 44 completed medical forms could be found. Of the remainder, either the child refused a medical, or the medical forms could not be traced in the social services' records.

Of the completed forms reviewed, few were completed in any detail. Immunization status was completed in less than 50%, and only two-thirds of these gave full details, including dates. Growth in height was measured in 91% and weight in 80%, but less than a third gave centiles, and only one or two had centile charts attached despite both these being specifically requested on the forms. Physical examination was completed, but only 20% tested and recorded visual acuity using a recognized test. Only 4.5% tested hearing using a recognized hearing test. Several examples of hearing testing using a 'tuning fork' or 'spoken voice' were cited. Less than a quarter gave any detail about development, behaviour, or general recommendations on treatment or follow up required.

As carried out at present, the medical is potentially dangerous as chronic conditions may be present that need ongoing treatment and follow up, but in the absence of a medical history the child may be given a falsely reassuring 'clean bill of health'.

Problems of care services for 'looked after' children

Despite the guidelines of the Children Act, there remain many problems with the care of 'looked after' children.

In his review, Sir William Utting (Children in the Public Care, 1991) noted the following problems:

1. Lack of participation by children in decisions affecting their lives
2. Lack of information about their rights
3. Haphazard process of health assessment
4. Use of medical services largely in response to illness
5. Little concern with prevention and health education
6. Lack of psychological and psychiatric support for children

Much of this was borne out by actually asking the young people themselves for their views about their medical care (Table 11.9).

The residential sector is now a service largely for adolescents. As a group, they are able to express their views about their health concerns and about the health care which is available to them. They have often missed health and sex education at school because of frequent changes of school and non-attendance. Many have little information about their own medical history.

The children are ostensibly protected by the statutory requirement for an annual medical examination, but many default as they become older. It may be that they do not perceive a rigid timetable of physical examinations as

Table 11.9   Young people's views on the current system of medical examination

---

These were recently sought in six community homes
Comments and suggestions included:
   'I feel I am not listened to'
   'I don't like them'
   'No more please'
   'I wish the doctor would talk to me and not my keyworker all the time'
   'Pathetic. Didn't do anything. Need more information from the doctor. Don't tell you what's going on'
   'Take more notice'
   'We should be allowed to go with someone we feel safe with'
   'Privacy. Given more information. Choice of doctor male or female. More often when needed'
In contrast, only one child made a positive comment: 'They are good'

---

relevant to their health needs. Problems and worries do not occur to coincide with the annual medical!

The current system is not meeting the real health needs of the children. As adolescents, they need to learn how to access health care when they feel they need it, and to develop trust in the health professionals they deal with. They also need to be able to start independent life with a good basic knowledge of health and sexual health issues. The processes of assessment and ongoing management of health of this group of young people urgently needs reviewing if it is to offer a service in line with the letter and spirit of the Children Act.

Regular visits to community homes by interested health professionals, perhaps mainly an appropriately trained school nurse and possibly a family planning nurse, would be likely to achieve more in terms of health education, trust, and a reasonably rapid response to queries and concerns as they arise, than annual physical examinations. They would have the added benefit of easy access to further medical advice, and could be used as a means of informing and updating the community homes staff on health issues and local services.

The purposes for which information about the health of the child and his or her family is collected are complex. They include the following:

1. The need for Social Services to plan and provide for the care of the child
2. The documentation of the physical and emotional status of the child for medico-legal reasons. This may be used to prepare a case to provide evidence for the courts to remove the child from his parents, and also to protect the prospective carers from future allegations of failing to care for the child
3. The child's own future reference and information in later life
4. Research into the health needs of this group of children, including evaluation of preventative aspects of their care

A review by the Department of Health of current research about child placement and their outcomes (Patterns and Outcomes in Child Placement) concluded that social workers have a complex task in obtaining information, accurate recording and organization of this information, careful analysis, and weighing up the evidence so produced in order to meet these needs as fully as possible. Health was recommended as one of the 7 outcomes to be assessed. Many placements break down at an alarming rate, and these children, who are in desperate need of stability in their lives, can be moved several times in a short time. Good record keeping is particularly important in these cases to ensure some continuity in their care. However, the complexity of the task, the difficulties of corporate parenting, and the resources available may all combine to make the ideal very difficult to achieve.

It is easy to be critical of the work of residential social workers, but this must be understood against the background of their having in their charge some of the most 'difficult' children in our society, and that up to 60% of them are untrained. It certainly seems very difficult for the outsider to appreciate this. It is rather like the pre-registration house-physician being given responsibility for the care of patients with the most complex medical problems. There are, of course, more senior field social work staff and more senior staff within the care system, but staff shortages and staff turnover can often leave the residential social workers with insufficient guidance or support.

Residential social workers work a shift system, and therefore in the residential home, children have a confusing array of people to deal with. A residential home with 15 children will have around 15 staff, one of whom will be the young person's key worker, who will be around for some, but not all, of the week. There will also be a social worker in the area team that is managing the young person's 'case', and often contact with parents and other family members.

It is difficult forming relationships in what is a network rather than a family. The other young people have usually suffered similar emotional problems, and in some homes there is a considerable turnover in the young people residing there as well as the staff in attendance. The picture is completed by the bleak and bare furnishings and state of disrepair in some (but happily far from all) residential homes.

The doctor who is providing the report cannot provide really useful advice without knowledge of the individual community home, just as one of the strengths of our primary health care teams is knowledge of the individual children registered with the practice.

The problems of high staff turnover in the residential care setting and the more general problems of corporate parenting are compounded by lack of training of residential care staff in many key areas of their work.

A pilot study in Nottingham compared the knowledge of parents with that of residential social workers about common health problems and their management of particular situations, for example a child with a fever or a child who does not want to eat. We will not present the detailed results here. However, among the marks awarded on this short test, all the highest scores for correct answers were ordinary parents and all of the bottom scorers were residential social workers. There were, of course, wide variations in knowledge between both groups. Incorrect answers were graded into harmless (i.e. measures that will not help but will not cause damage), and potentially harmful (i.e. practices that are not only ineffective but whose implementation would carry extra risks for the child). Both residential social workers and parents gave dangerous answers to many of the questions.

This short questionnaire led us to identify the need to train residential social workers (and parents) in a wide range of issues relating to health care, health promotion and mental health.

The main headings for this training are listed below:

A	Child health surveillance	I	Sexual behaviour, pregnancy and sexually transmitted disease
B	Immunization and infection		
C	Common illnesses	J	Drugs: legal, illegal, prescribed, non-prescribed, including tobacco
D	Growth and development		
E	Emotional development		
F	Use of health services	K	Families, cycles of deprivation
G	Diet	L	Conduct disorders
H	Accident prevention and first aid	M	Depression

Another major problem is the general lack of awareness amongst other professional groups about what the health services overall, and Community Paediatrics in particular, have to offer. There is a lack of definition of the roles of different individuals. The scope of 'the medical' for coordinating health care rather than a one-off physical examination is greatly underestimated and undervalued.

The Audit Commission, in their report *'Seen but not heard'* (1994), was critical of the current situation and stressed the need for improvement. They emphasized the need for residential care to be carefully planned, with set objectives, regularly reviewed by professionals involved, and with close liaison between Social Services, Health and Education, to ensure maximum support for the young person.

The Children Act has given us specific recommendations with statutory obligations towards the care of all 'looked after' children, and young people in residential homes are an extremely vulnerable subgroup of these with very special needs to be met.

In order to enable this to happen, community paediatricians need to look very carefully at the service that is currently available to young people in residential homes in their districts, and how this can be developed to meet the needs of this group of 'children in need'.

THE WAY FORWARD

The Children Act guidelines leave both local authorities and health authorities with definite, statutory requirements for the optimal care of young people in residential homes.

Young people, mainly adolescents, in residential care are a very special group of children who require a separate programme of care, rather than simply being included within the services developed for all children. The contract for this programme, which comes under the general umbrella of 'children in need', must include a service specification for comprehensive assessment and on-going management in the fields of general health care, including and emphasizing mental health and health promotion.

Community paediatricians have a very important and difficult task in coordinating health care for 'looked after' children. They need to secure with local authorities workable agreements for providing support, including general medical care in the widest sense, and also including psychological and psychiatric support and health promotion. They may need to act as advocates, both locally and nationally, for this group of very needy young people. One or more senior paediatricians should have a designated role in each district to ensure that this is addressed.

They need to ensure that the procedures for notification of a child entering care are in place and are effective in practice.

The initial medical assessment of the child looked after should be viewed as an ongoing collation of health related information over a period of time, rather than a one off 'medical'.

The key worker in social services responsible for the care of the child should gain some understanding of the nature of a comprehensive medical assessment, and should be asked to collect together as much information about the child's history as possible before the first medical appointment. Ideally, special forms should be designed for this, and their use and significance agreed and adhered to.

Careful consideration is needed about who carries out the medical assessment, what training and experience is needed, what forms are used to record the information, and how this information is subsequently stored and used so as to be most directly useful for the care of the young person.

A health care plan should be produced and used actively to contribute to the overall care plan for the young person at statutory reviews. The young people themselves must be actively and directly involved in all of this process, and be encouraged to participate in making plans for the future.

Ongoing health care to young people in residential homes can be provided optimally by designated health professionals linked to community homes, with appropriate expertise to deal with these very vulnerable young people. These children need specific health care time allocated to them via a specialized service designed to meet both their routine and exceptional needs.

All the health professionals involved should aim to become known to, and trusted by, both young people and staff of residential homes. They will need to make links with local primary health care teams, and liaise with school health services generally. There is also a need to develop a wide network of health professionals, including child and adolescent psychiatry, clinical psychology, health promotion, genitourinary specialists, and family planning services, who would work together to provide on-going support to community homes.

Links would ideally be set up with a wide range of support organizations, including voluntary, such as hostels for homeless young people, and support organizations for abuse victims.

It would also be important to develop close liaison with education to try to ensure attendance and satisfactory progress in school, meeting special educational needs, effective management of emotional and behavioural problems, and full involvement in school life.

Regular visits to community homes by interested health professionals, and perhaps using appropriately trained school nurses to develop surveillance and health promotion programmes within the homes, as well as supplying regular opportunities for consultation, both to young people and staff, would greatly improve the service offered to community homes from the health service.

Ideally, there should be continuity in this so that both the residents themselves and the staff could build up relationships and mutual trust. Individual homes could be encouraged to include programmes of health education and health care in their statements of objectives.

The availability of health care to young people on the streets and involved in prostitution is even more difficult to improve. To move forward, a multi-disciplinary approach is essential. Both prevention and intervention strategies need to be developed. There is scope for innovation to help these vulnerable children.

Firstly   Child prostitutes must be considered as victims of child abuse and not criminals, and this needs to be reflected in guidance issued by Area Child Protection Committees, the Department of Health and the Home Office.

Secondly   We should consider targeting therapeutic and supportive services to prevent families rejecting their abused children, and to support the emotional needs of rejected children.

Thirdly   The interventions offered to young people involved in prostitution should be made available to them in ways which they can accept. For example, in our area the genitourinary clinic has links with Prostitute Outreach Workers (POW). These are ex-prostitutes who advise and support prostitutes and link them into services. It has been more difficult to access under-age girls, so a recent development is the appointment of a young worker to link with young girls and an ex-rent boy to make links with male sex workers.

Lastly   There needs to be research in this country to look at the extent of juvenile prostitution here, and to examine the needs of this population of young people, with reference to culture, sexuality, and disability.

The regular statutory medical reviews of 'looked after' children, which remain a requirement by law under the Children Act could perhaps be used to focus on updating the health care plan, and contributing to the statutory reviews by social services. It has also been suggested that an annual report on the health of individuals, and of the community home itself, could be produced as information that would assist in the longer term planning of services.

The development of some form of child held records, e.g. 'my health passport' or the national parent-held record modified for school age children, would enable the passing on of information, including when the young person leaves care. Some medical involvement on leaving care, whether to own family or independent living, giving young people and/or their carer written information about their health, past and family history, immunizations, results of surveillance.

Community paediatricians may need to have some direct involvement in ongoing support and training of staff, and in coordinating health promotion services for the young people, both in groups and on an individual, one-to-one basis.

All of this would require the setting up and maintenance of good information systems relating to 'looked after' children. There needs to be good communication, both at a strategic level and in day-to-day work, with effective and regularly reviewed networks.

Community paediatricians may well feel the need to raise the profile of these problems both with other health professionals and with purchasers.

They may also see a need for on-going involvement with social services in developing preventative strategies, to minimize family breakdown and inability of parents to look after their children.

Evaluation of these aspects of community paediatric work is important to ensure optimal development of the service to meet the highly complex needs of this very vulnerable group of youngsters.

There remains ample scope in the future for ongoing research and audit in this previously rather neglected area of paediatrics.

KEY POINTS FOR CLINICAL PRACTICE

- Young people in residential homes are a vulnerable and needy group from a multiply deprived background, and with a high risk of poor outcome.
- The majority are adolescents.
- They need a specialized medical service designed to identify and meet their routine and exceptional needs and to help them access appropriate health services.

- There is a statutory requirement for comprehensive assessment of physical and mental health, including immunizations, smoking, drugs, alcohol, sex, and the need for information and counselling about health matters.
- The young person needs to be actively involved and take part in all parts of this programme, which needs to address and be sensitive to issues related to gender, race, religion, disability, and sexual orientation.
- Comprehensive assessment should lead to the formulation of a health care plan which the young person 'owns'. This should be incorporated in the overall care plan for the young person, and actively followed and checked at Social Services reviews. This requires allocation of time, resources and real commitment.
- There needs to be, whenever possible, continuity of care — named personnel: medical, nursing, psychological, psychiatric, and family planning staff. Medical staff should have appropriate qualifications and experience in the care of children and young people, and access to all relevant medical records and family history.
- There is a need for ongoing training and support on a wide range of health related issues for staff working in a residential care setting.
- It is important to develop collaboration between health and social services such that clear policies are agreed and effectively carried out.
- Health services for these special young people need a system of evaluation.
- Community paediatricians need to be pro-active, raising the profile of these issues, and making a case for purchasers.

REFERENCES

1 Wolkind S N. Child placement. Driven by belief rather than research. Leader in BMJ. BMJ 1991; 303: 483
2 Bebbington A, Miles J. The background of children who enter local authority care. Br J Social Work 1989; 19(5): 349–368
3 Wedge P, Phelan J. Essex Child Care Survey 1981–1985. Social Work Development Unit, University of East Anglia, Norwich, 1987
4 Kahan B. Growing up in Care. Oxford: Blackwell, 1989
5 Kahan B. (ed) for the Open University. Child Care Research, Policy and Practice. Hodder and Stoughton, 1989
6 Essen J et al. School attainment of children who have been in care. Child Care Health Dev 1976; 2: 339–351
7 Heath A et al. The educational progress of children in and out of care. Br J Social Work 1989; 19: 447–460
8 Wolkind S, Rutter M. Women who have been 'in care' — psychological and social status during pregnancy. J Child Psychol Psychiatry 1977; 18: 179–182
9 Rutter M et al. In: Madge N, ed. Families at risk. Parenting in two generations: looking backwards and looking forwards. Heinemann, 1983
10 Wolkind S, Rutter M. Children who have been 'in care' — an epidemiological study. J Child Psychol Psychiatry 1973; 14: 97–105
11 Akhurst BA. The prevalence of behaviour problems among children in care. Educational Res 1975; 17(2): 137–142
12 Keane A. Behaviour problems among long-term foster children. Adoption and Fostering 1983; 7(3): 53–62
13 Lambert L et al. Variations in behaviour ratings of children who have been in care.

J Child Psychol Psychiatry 1977; 18: 335–346
14 Hendriks JH. The health needs of young people in care. Adoption and Fostering 1989; 13(1): 43–50
15 Simms M. The health surveillance of children in care — are there serious problems? Adoption and Fostering 1988; 12(4): 20–23
16 Robinson R. Children in care need better health care. Leader in BMJ. BMJ 1991; 302: 1293

KEY REPORTS

Bamford FN, Jepson A, Nourse CH. British Paediatric Association, Report of Working Party on Children in Care. December 1982
Report of the House of Commons Social Services Committee (Renee Short, Chairman). HMSO, 1984
DHSS SSI Inspection of Community Homes, 1985
Bamford F, Wolkind SN. The Physical and Mental Health of Children in Care: Research Needs. Economic and Social Research Council, 1988
Simms M. Health Surveillance Procedures for Children in Care. Institute for Social Studies in Medical Care, London. (Personal Communication)
Oxtoby M (ed). Children in Care: The Medical Contribution. BAAF, 1988
Parker RA. In: Sinclair (ed). Residential Care: The Research Reviewed. Residential Care for Children. HMSO/NISW, 1988
The Children Act 1989: Guidance and Regulations. Vol 3 and 4, HMSO, 1990
Department of Health. Patterns and Outcomes in Child Placement: Messages from Current Research and their Implications. HMSO, 1991
Department of Health Working Party Report. Assessing Outcomes in Child Care. HMSO, 1991
Utting W. Children in the Public Care. HMSO, 1991
Choosing with Care. Report of Committee of Enquiry. Chaired by Norman Warner. HMSO, 1992
Health and Personal Social Services Statistics for England. HMSO, 1993
Bullock R, Little M, Millham S. Residential Care for Children: A Review of the Research. HMSO, 1993
Woodroffe C et al. Children, Teenagers and Health — The Key Data Open University Press, 1993
Children Act Report 1993. HMSO, 1994
Audit Commission Report. Seen but not heard. HMSO, 1994

12. Commissioning health services for adolescents

A. Macfarlane

This chapter concerns the commissioning and purchasing of health/medical services for people aged 10–18 years. The justification for looking at the commissioning issues as they concern this age group is that frequently their care falls between many different providers. These include the adolescents themselves, their parents, the primary health care team, the community and the hospital paediatric services and the adult services. Where their care is provided by the professionals working within the National Health Service (NHS) there may be a lack of clear responsibility for ensuring the appropriateness (in terms of both quantity and quality) of the services provided for them in the wide and increasingly fragmented structures that go to make up the present NHS.

This fragmentation can be overcome by the commissioners/purchasers of adolescent services (including the district health authorities, the family health services authorities, and organizations representing non-fundholding and fundholding GPs) and the providers of adolescent services, together developing an overall district-wide strategy for these services. This can then be used in the contractual processes between purchasers and providers (particularly in defining the quality issues), for when the providers develop their business plans, and for developing appropriate facilities in primary health care.

A further use of a strategy is that it can begin to clarify what is usefully (effectively) supplied by the health services and what is best supplied outside of the health services. This applies to allied services such as social and education services, but much more particularly it applies to aspects of adolescent health which are dependent on national political policies relating to factors, such as employment, and social and economic equality. These are the direct responsibility of the government. Health professionals, whether in the purchaser or provider field, although having to take account of these factors should never allow themselves to be seen as being able to adequately compensate for ineffective and inadequate political policies.

It is the aim of this chapter to aid in the development of such a strategy for adolescent services that can be agreed between purchasers and providers.

BACKGROUND INFORMATION FOR PURCHASING HEALTH SERVICES FOR ADOLESCENTS

One of the major problems of purchasing services for adolescents (as in many other areas of purchasing) is the lack of precise information. Because various sources of information give different age breakdowns, the information below does not always cover the age group defined, but it does give some idea of present national mortality, morbidity and service usage. In most cases the figures given are those for England and Wales.

Mortality

In 1992, out of a total of 1922 deaths in the 10–19-year age group in England and Wales, 1021 (53%) were due to injury or poisoning, with the second most common reason, neoplasms, only accounting for 14% (Fig. 12.1). The third most common cause of death was diseases of the nervous system, the fourth was diseases due to respiratory problems.

Morbidity and use of services

The General Household Survey of 1992 found that in 5–15-year-olds 19% of males and 18% of females rated themselves as having a long-standing illness. In the same age group, 9% of males and 10% of females reported themselves as having restricted activity (Table 12.1). Further data from the General Household Survey[1] shows that, on average, young people visit their GP three or four times a year. The reasons for these visits are shown by the OPCS figures for 1991/1992 for GP consultation rates for children aged 5–14/15 and 15/16–24. These are shown in Fig. 12.2, with respiratory diseases being far the most common.

Levels of reported attendance at outpatients or casualty for the 5–15-year-olds in 1992 was 12% in males and 10% in females.[1] Detailed data about

Table 12.1 Trends in self-reported sickness in persons aged 5–15: percentage of persons reporting long-standing illness and restricted activity

Great Britain	1979	1980	1981	1982	1983	1984	1985	1986	1987	1988	1989	1990	1991	1992
Long-standing illness														
Males	14		15		18		19		20	20	17		19	
Females	10		13		13		15		16	17	15		18	
Restricted activity														
Males	11		11		11		13		12	11	11		9	
Females	11		11		12		14		13	13	9		10	

Source: General Household Survey 1992.

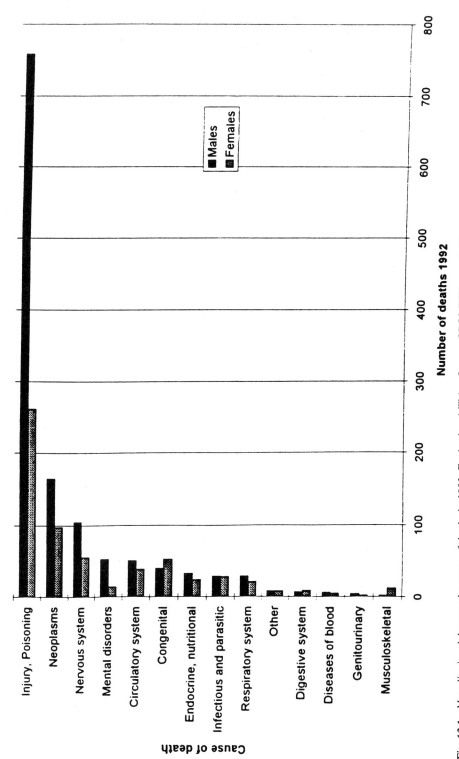

Fig. 12.1 Mortality in adolescents by cause of death, in 1992, England and Wales. Source: OPCS DH2 nos. 9, 19.

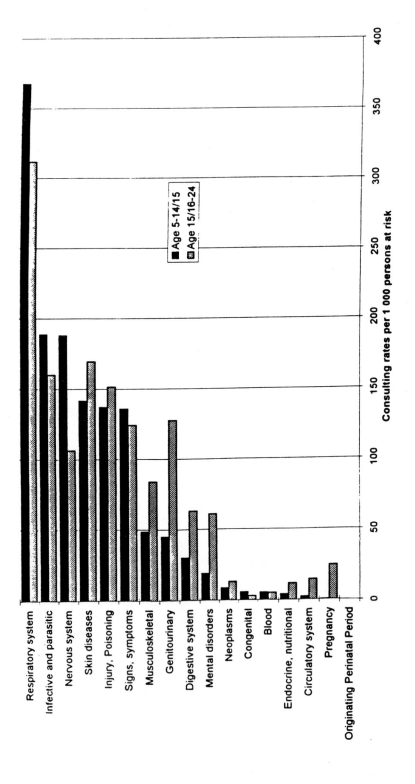

Fig. 12.2 GP consultations. Patient consulting rates by category 1991/1992, ages 5–24, England and Wales. Source: OPCS MSGP 4 1991/2.

hospital admission can be obtained by looking at the data from the Oxford record linkage study.[2] At 10 years, 22% of hospital admissions were to general paediatrics, 24% to general surgery, 23% to ear nose and throat surgery and 20% to trauma and orthopaedics. By 14 years of age, only 6% of general hospital paediatric admissions were to general paediatrics. By 16 years of age 24% of hospital admissions for girls were to gynaecology and less than 1% to general paediatrics, and 40% of admissions of young men were to trauma and orthopaedics. The most common cause for admission in young men was head injury; termination of pregnancy was the single most common reason for admission of girls aged 15 and 16 years. Self-poisoning was also common amongst older teenage girls. Most admissions of adolescents are therefore for surgical rather than for medical reasons and are for problems influenced by behavioural factors rather than disease processes.

Dental health has greatly improved in recent years and the proportion of 15-year-olds entirely free of dental caries has risen from 8% in 1983 to 40% in 1993.[3]

Mental health problems, defined as abnormalities of behaviour or social relationships sufficiently marked or prolonged to cause suffering or risk to optimal development and sufficiently severe to be disabling, have been found to occur in 2.4% of all children up to the age of 16 in Great Britain. It is higher in the adolescent age group than in younger children.

Health-related behaviours in adolescents

Smoking

The most up-to-date national data on smoking in teenagers in England comes from the Schools Health Education Unit at the University of Exeter.[4] Their eighth report 'Young people in 1993' contains data on 29 074 young people aged 11–16 years. In broad terms, by the age of 16, one-third of teenagers will never have smoked, one-third will have tried and given up and one-third will be smoking either regularly or occasionally. The smoking rate is not reducing in this age group.

Alcohol

The age of initiation of alcohol use is getting younger — presently standing at 10–11 years. Early initiates usually report heavier drinking later in adulthood. Studies show that teenagers are more likely to have casual sex and less likely to use a condom when under the influence of alcohol. There is a strong association between alcohol use and stress and coping difficulties in adolescents. Many adolescents who overdose do so while under the influence of alcohol. Longitudinal studies suggest that drinking per se in adolescence does not predict drinking patterns in adulthood, but that certain drinking patterns in adolescents such as frequent drunkenness, early initiation, drinking mainly in public houses does predict serious alcohol problems in adulthood.[5]

Sex

The median age of first sexual experience (any experience of a sexual kind — for example, kissing, cuddling, petting) has dropped over the last four decades from 16 to 14 for women and from 15 to 13 for men. The median age of first intercourse over the same period of time has dropped from 19 to 17 in men and from 20 to 17 in women. Amongst 16–24-year-olds, 2.7% of women and 9.3% of men report having experienced intercourse before the age of 15, and 33.8% of women and 55.8% of men reported having some sexual experience before this age. By the age of 16 (the age of consent) 18.7% of women and 27.6% of men had had intercourse. Although 'non-use' of contraception at first intercourse has declined over recent decades, even today, when first intercourse occurs before the age of 16, nearly half of young women and over half of young men report using no method either being used by themselves or by their partners.[6]

Drugs

A cohort of 776 14- and 15-year-olds attending eight schools across the north-west of England are currently being followed using self-reporting questionnaires, and ensuring complete confidentiality. Respondents were asked two questions relating to illegal drugs, solvents and magic mushrooms: whether they had ever been around when the drugs were offered and whether they had ever tried them. Fifty-nine per cent had been offered at least one drug. Cannabis had been offered to 52% of all children, LSD to 36%, amphetamines to 26%, solvents to 22%, magic mushrooms to 21%, nitrites to 21%, methylene-dioxy-methamphetamine (MDMA) (Ecstasy) to 18%. Seven per cent had been in situations where cocaine was offered and 4% where heroine was available. In the majority of cases where drugs were offered they had not been accepted, but 6 out of 10 offered a drug had tried at least one at some time. Thirty-six per cent of the entire sample of 14–15-year-olds had tried at least one drug.[7] Other studies further south have confirmed that this study does appear to be representative of present drug exposure and drug taking in England and Wales.

The range of services for adolescents

It is sometimes difficult to conceptualize the number of different services within the NHS supplied to this age group, and below is an attempt at a reminder of all the services, apart from adolescents themselves, and their parents, that may deliver such services. These are listed in Table 12.2.

Table 12.2   Services supplied for adolescents within the NHS

— Services provided by the primary health care team
— Family planning services supplied by the community
— Community services covering adolescents with other 'special needs' and for adolescents 'in need'
— Services covering child protection work
— Community dental services
— School health services
— Other community services including, speech therapy, physiotherapy, occupational therapy
— Public health medicine services including infectious disease control and health promotion, particularly those concerning the 'health of the nation' targets
— Paediatric and adult services for mental health care
— Services for adolescents with learning difficulties
— Secondary and tertiary paediatric medical services
— Secondary and tertiary adult medical services
— Secondary and tertiary general paediatric surgical services
— Secondary and tertiary adult surgical services
— Secondary and tertiary orthopaedic services
— Ear, nose and throat services
— Neurosurgery
— Plastic surgery
— Ophthalmological services
— Accident and emergency facilities
— Traumatology
— Gynaecological services
— Maternity services
— Anaesthesiology

Needs assessment for adolescents

With the present funding of the NHS, 'needs assessment' will realistically always have to be relatively unsophisticated and 'quick and dirty'. This is because (1) there is a lack of routinely collected relative information, (2) it is impossible to totally meld together the various 'needs' as perceived by the adolescents themselves, their parents, politicians, social services, education services, public health services, other doctors, nurses, managers, etc., (3) there is no method of setting priorities for these 'needs' once they are agreed, (4) there is a gross lack of resources to meet these needs once they are both agreed and prioritized.

Purchasing priority should, however, be given to ensuring that there is a minimum data set for the district which is reliable and covers age-appropriate information concerning:

— data from accident and emergency departments concerning accidents and injuries
— acute morbidity data from primary, secondary and tertiary care

— chronic morbidity data concerning adolescents with chronic diseases and adolescents with impairments, disabilities and handicaps
— data concerning lifestyles of adolescents which are relative to their present health, and to future health outcomes
— data concerning adolescents with learning difficulties and/or emotional and behavioural disturbances.

Data about 'perceived needs' of parents of adolescents and of the adolescents themselves are best carried out on an 'as needed' basis, using sampling techniques amongst suitably representative populations.

OVERALL PURCHASING PRINCIPLES FOR ADOLESCENT HEALTH SERVICES

Because health service provision for adolescents is so diffuse between various departments, units, trusts and levels of care, a core set of 'purchasing principles' is essential. Table 12.3 shows one suggested set.

PURCHASING AND PROVIDING PRIMARY HEALTH CARE SERVICES FOR ADOLESCENTS

Whatever else, it is essential that the services supplied by the primary health care services are seen as 'user friendly' by adolescents. To achieve this needs little in the way of resources and could include the following:

— Identifying the characteristics of a practice's 10–18-year-old population by using the practice's age/sex register and using a degree of common sense and the primary health care team's knowledge of local factors.
— Providing positive information about confidentiality. Research shows[8] that this is the single most important issue as seen by adolescents. They do not know or assume that their discussions with members of the primary health care team will be treated with absolute confidentiality, and this fact needs to be positively advertised to them.
— Making the practice more adolescent user friendly. A priority should be to make sure that the GPs themselves, practice nurses and the receptionists are user friendly to adolescents (not always easy to achieve).
— Providing telephone advice to adolescents on a non-named basis. This facility is rated second only to confidentiality by teenagers and needs to be positively advertised to them.[8]
— Offering freedom to change GP at the age of 16. Practices should consider sending a note to all those in their practice population reaching the age of 16 explaining what services the practice has to offer them and that they can choose to go to any GP they wish.
— Routine checks at 16 years of age may be one way of helping to contact adolescents and providing them with information about practice services. Some research supports this concept.[9]

Table 12.3   Purchasing principles for adolescent services

- Commissioning for adolescents (as for children) should always be part of a comprehensive overall strategy which includes services supplied by primary health care, social services, education, and voluntary organizations, as well as services supplied by community health services, and hospitals services; such a strategy should be drawn up by all those involved
- Adolescents themselves should be consulted about their health needs and involved in the development of medical services provided for them
- It is essential for the mental and physical well-being of adolescents and their parents that health promotion and prevention should always be considered alongside treatment
- Commissioning of services for adolescents should be information-based, reflect the needs of the local population (single parent families, homeless, ethnic groups), be flexible enough to respond to the needs of a rapidly changing population and should avoid unnecessary duplication whilst taking into account tertiary services also provided by trusts to populations beyond the boundaries of the commissioning authority
- Services for adolescents should be free at the time of delivery and adhere to the basic principles of 'equity' central to the NHS
- Adolescent and family mental health should be considered alongside physical health at all stages of commissioning
- Adolescents should be fully involved with, consulted about, and informed about their health by health professionals working in partnership with them
- Emphasis should be put on the development of ambulatory care for adolescents and they are only admitted to hospital when the care they require cannot equally well be provided in other ways; family circumstances, parental wishes and need for social support must, however, be taken into account.
- With all health and illness services supplied for adolescents (e.g. emergency, obstetrics, ear, nose and throat, dental, eyes, mental health, dermatology, sexually transmitted disease clinics, etc.), adolescents should enjoy the care of appropriately trained staff with suitable communication skills, using effective interventions, in environments appropriate for their age and understanding
- The training of all health professionals caring for adolescents has quality standards and resource implications that must be included in the commissioning process
- Commitment to 'joint commissioning' of services between health, social services and education for adolescents should be sought for work, including: child protection (Working Together under the Children Act 1989, HMSO, 1991), adolescents with special needs (Education Act 1993), adolescents in need (Children Act 1989), school health (Services for School Age Children – British Paediatric Association 1994), and health promotion ('health of the nation' HMSO, 1992)
- Quality standards, critical evaluation of effectiveness, methods of monitoring and measurement of outcomes should be decided on by discussion between the providers and commissioners

---

- Clinics specifically for adolescents. These are beginning to be set up by many practices all over the UK but their effectiveness has not been evaluated.
- Specific help and information for parents to help them in their role as primary carers of their children. During most of the teenage years, parents continue to be the main providers, carers and source of information, and this role could be more fully recognized by those providing primary health care.

PURCHASING COMMUNITY CARE FOR ADOLESCENTS

These purchasing issues cover a wide range of statutory provision as well as other health services responsive to the needs of adolescents.

Children 'in need' and the Children Act 1989

The needs met under the Children Act are:

— the need of the child/adolescent to have his/her welfare seen as paramount
— the need for a child/adolescent to be bought up in a happy, secure and safe environment.

Some of the services that need to be purchased to meet these needs include:

— the examination of adolescents suspected of being abused/neglected
— attendance of health professionals at case conferences
— providing reports and attending court cases (other than criminal proceedings where expenses are paid by the court system)
— services to supply the medical and health services required under the appropriate statutes to meet the health needs of adolescents in care
— the early identification of adolescents 'in need'
— to fulfil the obligation to notify the local authority of accommodated adolescents
— for all staff to know the district child protection policies and how they apply to adolescents and to act on them appropriately.

The Education Act 1993

The needs met under the Education Act 1993 are:

— the need for children's/adolescents' special educational needs to be identified as early as possible
— the need for parents to be involved in the provision of resources to help their child
— the need for children with special needs and their parents to be provided with a coordinated provision from all the services concerned.

The purchasers need to commission services that:

— aid the identification and notification to the education authorities of children with 'special needs'
— carry out medical examinations and submit the reports for the multiprofessional assessments requested by the education services within specified time limits
— carry out further assessments as requested by the education authorities.

Adolescents with health and developmental problems

The needs for children with disabilities and their families are:

— the need for early identification of the problem
— the need for a diagnosis of the problem
— the need for appropriate, coordinated and effective management, treatment and overall care.

Purchasers need to commission services that:

— ensure the early identification of all children/adolescents with disabilities living within the district and providing the necessary support, management and treatment to the child and their family
— provide health/medical care of children/adolescents in secondary schools.

Health promotion and primary prevention services supplied by the community child health services relative to adolescents

— appropriate immunization of all adolescents in the population
— promoting the use of cycle helmets
— providing factual information about smoking, drugs, alcohol, contraception, exercise, diet
— family planning services.

Other purchasing issues relative to the community child health services for adolescents

— communication between professionals within the child health services and outside the health services
— continuing support for teaching and research, although where the budget for these activities should come from is still not clear
— promoting audit and 'in service' training
— the need for health professionals to be involved in management and administration
— services for children with disabilities aged 16–19 years.

PURCHASING AND PROVIDING HOSPITAL CARE FOR ADOLESCENTS

Some purchasing quality issues raised by Action for Children in Hospital[10] are:

— where possible there should be separate accommodation within adult or children's wards, including space for socialization and homework, but because in average district general hospitals the number of medical wards may be small, separate facilities may not be practical

— any facilities that are developed for adolescents need the involvement of the adolescents themselves in the design and decoration
— the provision of appropriate facilities for their needs, particularly concerning privacy, bed size, appropriate decoration, magazines, access to television, reasonable hours for having to be in bed, etc.
— involving adolescents in their own treatment
— encouraging visits from family and friends
— a generalist paediatric consultant with a special interest in the problems of adolescents
— training of nursing and other staff to deal with the specific needs of adolescents
— appropriate information which has been developed with adolescents themselves
— flexibility in organization of ward life, such as allowing 'take away' food to be brought in.

Purchasing transition of care to adult services

This is an area of purchasing which is still developing because:

— services have to be flexible as to when the care of adolescents with health needs is handed over from the paediatric/child health services to adult services
— there is need to take account of the needs of the individual adolescent, the type of service being provided, the locality and the nature and abilities of the professionals involved
— the overall strategy should ensure that local principles for transfer are identified, in place, and actioned in all the various services covered.

PURCHASING SERVICES FOR ADOLESCENTS WITH MENTAL HEALTH PROBLEMS

In purchasing services for the needs of adolescents with mental health problems, the following considerations need to be taken into account:[11]

— the level and type of current mental health porblems in children and young people
— the services of known benefit from the scientific and professional point of view
— the requirements of children and their families and carers
— the interests of local people, GPs, providers and their clinical staff, local authorities, family health service authorities and NHS management executive.

PURCHASING FOR ADOLESCENTS WITH LEARNING DIFFICULTIES

There are a number of major purchasing issues in this area which need further work at local and national level. These purchasing issues cannot normally be dealt with in isolation from services provided by the local education services and social services (see section on joint commissioning below). These issues include:

— evidence that more severely disabled children with learning difficulties are surviving into adolescence and their care needs begin to exceed those that can be provided by the family
— that changing service delivery patterns brought about by cuts in social service and education funding are putting increased strain on NHS resources
— the need to prioritize NHS resources to those areas of service delivery that have been shown to be effective (whether this is assessment, advice, training of others, etc.)
— consideration needs to be given to 'locality' provision of services.

JOINT COMMISSIONING OF SERVICES FOR ADOLESCENTS WITH SOCIAL SERVICES

Joint commissioning of services between health education and social services has become a major growth area. Although many of the problems have been identified, with shrinking resources it is essential that the services cooperate together with voluntary organizations at all levels of provision. These include:

— developing an overall strategy for commissioning that is needs based
— developing clearly defined roles for the immediate carers, health services, social services, education services
— recognizing where these roles overlap and cooperation has to occur
— the need for a joint protocol for purchasing equipment to support adolescents with special needs and their families
— the need to have a commonly shared register concerning all children and adolescents 'with special needs' between the three services
— agreements on meeting the statutory obligations under the Education Act, the Children Act, the Fostering and Adoption Regulations, regulations covering child protection work, in spite of the fact that this obligation ignores the limited resources available in the health services
— developing suitable information for adolescents with special needs, and their carers, concerning the services that are available
— developing 'healthy alliances' as part of the 'health of the nation' initiatives, that acknowledge the fact that the significant target to be met in the areas of diet, smoking, exercise, alcohol use, suicide, drugs

and unintended pregnancy are more dependent on government socio-economic policies than on service delivery in health, social services and education.

Quality issues concerning adolescent services

Many of the core quality issues are embodied in the 'purchasing principles' outlined in Table 12.3. The most essential two are:

— adolescents should be fully involved with, consulted about, and informed about their health by health professionals working in partnership with them
— with all health and illness services supplied for adolescents (e.g. paediatrics, emergency, obstetrics, ear, nose and throat, dental, eyes, mental health, dermatology, sexually transmitted disease clinics, etc.), adolescents should enjoy the care of appropriately trained staff with suitable communications skills, using effective interventions, in environments appropriate for their age and understanding.

Other quality issues will be specific to specific services and need to be developed at district level.

Effective purchasing for health promotion, and the 'health of the nation' initiatives for adolescents

Recent evidence indicates that many of the 'health of the nation' targets for adolescent health as outlined below are going to be difficult to achieve either by health services intervention or by forming healthy alliances. The reason is that the behaviours on which the mortality and morbidity depend appear to be due to factors beyond the control of the services concerned.

— Cutting the smoking rate of 11–15-year-olds by 33% — from 8% in 1989 to 6% (60% of adult smokers started before the age of 16). The only two major interventions that, on present evidence, will have an effect are increasing the price of cigarettes and banning cigarette advertising. The present NHS purchasing role should be to ensure that services are available to aid adolescents and young adults to give up smoking if they want to.
— Cutting the calories from fat — from 40% to below 35% of total calorie intake (eating habits are embedded even as far back as the womb, with the result of high cholesterol being laid down in the coronary arteries from an early age). It could be argued that there is a role for purchasing the provision of information by health professionals on an opportunistic basis, but the advice in this area changes not only over time, but also from one professional group to another.
— Cutting deaths due to accidents in the 15–24-year age group by 25% — from 23.2 per 100 000 to no more than 17.4 (the major cause of death

in young people). The role of purchasing here is uncertain as most deaths in this age group are male and are due to road traffic accidents. Opportunistically there may be a limited role for promoting the use of cycle helmet wearing.

— Cutting the pregnancy rate in girls under 16' by 50% — from 9.5 per 1000 girls aged 13–15 in 1989 to no more than 4.8 (pregnancy during the teens has a higher rate of prematurity and there is also a wide range of socioeconomic consequences). Here there is a definite role for purchasing the provision of contraceptive advice, especially in the area of emergency contraception in forms that meet the needs of adolescents.

— Cutting the overall suicide rate by 15% — from 11.1 per 100 000 population in 1990 to no more than 9.4 (there is a steady rise in male adolescent suicides at the present time). If the target is to be achieved, interventions are needed which are of proven effectiveness. However, review of available evidence offers little support for the aspiration that the posited targets can be achieved on the basis of current knowledge and current policy.

SOURCES OF INFORMATION OF EFFECTIVE INTERVENTIONS IN ADOLESCENT HEALTH USEFUL TO PURCHASERS

— The National Adolescent and Student Health Unit, Institute of Health Sciences, PO Box 777, Oxford, OX3 7LF
— The NHS Centre for Reviews and Dissemination, University of York, York, YO1 5DD
— The Institute of Health Policy Studies, Southampton University, Southampton, SOG 5NH
— The Health Education Association, Hamilton House, Mabledon Place, London, WC1H 9TX
— The Cochrane Centre, Summertown Pavillion, Middle Way, Oxford, OX2 7LG
— The Social Science Research Unit, Institute of Education, 18 Woburn Square, London, WC1H 0NS
— The Health Services Research Unit, University of Oxford, Department of Public Health and Primary Care, Gibson Building, Radcliffe Infirmary, Oxford, OX2 6HE
— The Health of Adolescents. In: On the state of the public health 1993, the annual report of the Chief Medical Officer of the Department of Health for the Year 1993. London: HMSO, 1995

REFERENCES

1 OPCS. General household survey 1992. London: HMSO, 1994
2 Henderson J, Goldacre M, Yeates D. Use of hospital in patient care in adolescence. Arch

Dis Child 1993; 69: 559–563

3 OPCS. Monitor SS/94/1, 1994
4 Balding J Young people in 1993. Schools Health Education Unit, University of Exeter
5 Swadi H. Alcohol abuse in adolescence: an update. Arch Dis Child 1993; 68: 341–343
6 Wellings K et al. Sexual behaviour in Britain: the nation survey of sexual attitudes and lifestyles. Harmondsworth: Penguin Books, 1994
7 Measham F, Newcome R, Parker H. The post-heroine generation. Druglink 1993; May/June 16–17
8 McPherson A, Macfarlane A. Promotion of the primary health care of adolescents in practice. (in press)
9 Donovan CF, McCarthy S. Is there a place for adolescent screening in general practice. Health Trends 1988; 20: 64
10 Setting standards for adolescents in hospital. London: Action for Children in Hospital, 1990
11 Kurtz Z, ed. With health in mind: mental health care for children and young people. London: Action for Sick Children, 1992

13. 'Born to fail' or 'Fit for the future'?

M. Manciaux, F.P. Debionne

Children who grow up in poverty or squalor, whose homes are grossly overcrowded, or who live in decaying inner-city neighbourhoods; children who are neglected or handicapped, or who are discriminated against on grounds of race, language, colour or religion; children whose parents are sick or psychiatrically disordered, who quarrel incessantly or who are absent: such children are in different ways 'disadvantaged'. They face greater odds than other children: they are more likely to suffer from physical illness or psychiatric disorder, or to fail educationally or to drop out of school or be 'early leavers', more likely to truant or become delinquent, or to leave school for unemployment or poorly skilled jobs.[1]

This quotation from the Court Report 'Fit for the future' is even more appropriate today than when it was written, 18 years ago. It is also quite pragmatic: 'the term [disadvantaged] has no precise meaning, but the implication is clear enough'.[1] Actually we have produced through the years a lot of papers, chapters of books, publications on children of the Fourth World,[2-6] based on a long association of one of us with Fourth World families. However, the recent developments of poverty, deprivation, social exclusion — of which children are the first and more vulnerable victims — pushes us to enlarge our approach to all children who are in jeopardy because their families are living in poverty, in difficulties of all kinds, in day-to-day survival which is a permanent struggle for a better future, apparently out of reach. And the current socioeconomic situation in our industrialized countries as well as some sociocultural changes have tended to increase dramatically the number of people living in such deleterious conditions.

Inequalities in the field of health, as a reflection of social inequalities, were documented as early as the first half of the nineteenth century, mainly in the industrializing European countries. One of the pioneers in this field was, in France, Villermé,[7] who published some observations that were really epidemiological, even before this word was ever used. Two of them are worth mentioning. While measuring young men who were living in Paris and had been called up for their military service, Villermé noticed marked differences in the height of the young recruits according to which part of Paris they came from. He deduced that the influence of poverty on growth is greater than that of climate. In 1840, he wrote, in an essay entitled 'La misère des ouvriers de l'industrie du coton': 'While in the families of manufacturers, merchants, drapers, directors of factories half the children reach the age of 29, this same half disappears before the age of two in the families of weavers and workers in cotton mills'. Thus he introduced the notion both of differential growth according to socioeconomic class and of differential mortality according to the socioprofessional status of the parents.

These inequalities (we would prefer the word 'inequities', which suggests 'iniquities', since they derive from an unfair social environment and management, and not from any genetic endowment) are being increasingly understood, and their study has led to a careful delineation of those factors that influence health, be they socioeconomic, sanitary, educational, cultural, professional, political. . . In fact, it is now well-known and acknowledged that inequities in the field of health are seldom isolated: they pertain to a vicious circle of cumulative handicaps (social disadvantages) which, by interaction, worsen the global picture. We shall see that it does not suffice to break this circle at one point — health for instance — to improve the situation of these children and families in poverty. However, before speaking of remedies and cure, let us consider first in some detail who these children in jeopardy are, what are the reasons for their poor condition and the repercussions on their health and future. For, as Mansel Prothero, speaking about malaria, wrote: 'An understanding of epidemiology requires a detailed knowledge of such things as the distribution of population, patterns of settlement, the nature of dwellings, administrative and social organization, and the range of the economic activities of those affected'.[8] The same wording could apply to the epidemiology of today's poverty: a clear definition of the population concerned and of its main characteristics is a prerequisite for any scientific and pragmatic approach, as well as for the planning of the necessary programmes.

CONCEPTUAL AND CONTEXTUAL APPROACH

In the period of global expansion following the Second World War (the so-called 'golden years of development' or, in France, 'the glorious thirties'), it was commonly thought and said that a mainstreaming process would progressively reduce and put an end to the remaining pockets of poverty in our industrialized countries and would, in turn, benefit the Third World. Even before the start of economic recession it became obvious that some groups, such as minorities, migrant workers and their families and also some indigenous families, were left behind in the socioeconomic growth. A monographic approach based on the methods of social anthropology helped identify the common characteristics of these groups: 'These are families from diverse ethnic backgrounds or origins, with long histories of social exclusion and extreme generational poverty. The outward signs of this exclusion as reflected in their handicaps are: low and irregular income; temporary housing (often without water and heat) or no housing at all; the absence of educational and vocational qualifications; ill health; and children who do not benefit from the educational system'.

Two major features emerge from this description: the transgenerational repetition — as if it were hereditary — and accumulation of basic insecurities in areas such as housing, income, employment, health. . . The first and lasting reaction of the privileged part of the population and, unfortunately, of too many health and social workers, was to accuse such people of laziness, inefficiency, if not of mental deficiency. The deprecatory term 'subculture of poverty' was even used, as if they had chosen to live in this precarious and marginal situation. Thanks to Joseph Wresinski, the founding father of the international movement ATD (Aide à Toute Détresse) Fourth World, and to his coworkers, a true partnership with these poor families has shown how things hang together to maintain them in their bad situation in spite of their willingness to escape from it. And the unethical victim-blaming process should continue no longer.

The 1970s brought, throughout the world, a growing economic turmoil with increasing unemployment, throwing into poverty millions of people in Western industrialized countries. Important and blunt social changes, such as the sharp increase in the participation of women in the labour force and the growing instability of marriages and families, have also influenced the fate of children in many ways.[10] The 'new poor' experience the same basic insecurities as Fourth World people, with additional handicaps: they are isolated, without the support that a movement such as ATD brings to its members.

At the beginning of the 1990s, the percentage of families with children in poverty varied, in the industrial world, 'between 4.5% in countries enjoying a highly developed system of social protection and 20% in countries with less developed social security';[10] the last figure applies to the USA. To speak only of the European scene, several factors have worsened the picture: a general trend to decentralization, with a progressive withdrawal of the State; the persistent economic crisis; the increasing number of one parent women-headed families with young children (the poorest part of the population in many societies); and, in Central and Eastern European countries, the collapse of the communist power. In this part of Europe, the proportion of poor children is certainly high, yet unknown.[11]

Clear evidence exists that relative inequality and poverty have increased in most industrialized countries over the last decade. The EC estimates that the number of people in poverty rose for its 12 member states from 38 million in 1975 to 44 million in 1985 and to 50 million in 1993 (i.e. 18% of the EC's population).[12] In the USA, from 1979 to 1987, the standard of living for the poorest fifth of the population fell by 9% while that of the top fifth rose by 9%. In global terms, the 1980s have witnessed a significant decline in human welfare and human capital formation in almost all of the industrialized world, a deepening of the gap between rich and poor, and a dramatic increase everywhere in the rate of unemployment.[10]

It is very difficult, however, to give precise figures concerning families and children living in poverty, because of the lack of a commonly agreed definition and because of the constantly evolving situation. This is why many authors make a plea for simple, yet accurate, 'markers' and why the EC, within the framework of its 'Poverty 3' programme, asks its member states to establish national observatories of social exclusion.[12]

Nevertheless, some national data are available, although they are difficult to compare from one country to another. In the UK, according to the National Children's Bureau: 'From 1979 to 1985, there was a 110% increase in children living in families dependent on supplementary benefit and a 25.7% increase in families with incomes below 50% of the average. In 1985, 3.5 million children were living in or on the margins of poverty'.[13] In France, 1 million family units (2.5 million persons) are living in great poverty. An additional 1.2 million families (3 million persons) are on the borders of financial precariousness.[14] In 1982, 5%, and in 1990, 7.5%, of children under 6 years of age were living in one parent families of which 92% were headed by a woman.[15] Various allowances are to some extent ameliorating the situation of these people left behind.[16] In the USA, one in four children under the age of 3 is poor; 14% of all children under 18 (and 27.5% of those below the poverty line) had no health insurance in 1990.[17] In Canada, in 1987, 15% of the population lived below the threshold of low income and 10% below the poverty line; for the women-headed one parent families, this latter index reaches 57%.[18]

One could go on with figures. What is more important is to identify as precisely as possible what the indicators of poverty are, some of them also being determinative factors. In his important report to the French Economic and Social Council and to the government (1987), Father Wresinski pointed to 'the accumulation of basic insecurities. . . which, according to their severity and duration, compromise a person's or family's ability to meet their responsibilities and enjoy their basic rights as citizens'.[19] Reported by Robbins,[20] the data of the EC poverty programmes show that children are affected in several ways: they are vulnerable to perinatal ill events, to poor health and nutrition, low school attainment, to being taken into the care of the state. For their part, young people are often early school leavers, entering into a range of training schemes that prolong childhood and make them dependent on parents and/or social assistance; they might then obtain some marginal employment and, on leaving their family, sometimes become homeless and enter into a poor adulthood. The report published in 1974 by the National Children's Bureau under the suggestive title 'Born to fail' is quite illustrative of this multiple handicap.[21] Multifactorial in its origin, poverty is multisectoral in its effects, and health is certainly one of the areas most affected.

CHILDREN'S HEALTH ENDANGERED

The association between poverty and childhood ill-health is now well documented not only in developing countries — where it assumes, through

the vicious circle of malnutrition/infection, an overwhelming importance —
but also in the most developed ones. Following Villermé,[7] the first evidence
came from disparities in life expectancy and differences in growth and
development between the well-to-do and the poor. Many epidemiological
surveys, some on a national scale, are now available and convincing. We shall
review a few of them, on specific topics.

Perinatal ill events

Preterm delivery and, to a lesser degree, low birth weight are closely
correlated with social class. The British perinatal survey,[22] as well as several
British studies reviewed by Spencer,[23] lead to the conclusion that 'this
correlation has been consistent over many years and various studies'. In
France, Papiernik introduced — as early as 1969 — a social class criterion in
his grid predictive of the risk of preterm delivery.[24] In Quebec, almost 10%
of infants born to disadvantaged mothers are small for dates.[25] Teenage
pregnancies, too closely spaced pregnancies, uncontrolled family size, perinatal ill events, and absence or shortness of breast feeding are more likely to
be found in underprivileged families. They represent at the same time the
consequences of unfavourable living conditions, and an increased risk of
perinatal or infant death and of child and maternal ill-health.

Developmental hazards

It is now well acknowledged that the growth and development of children
depend upon genetic, inherited factors, and on environmental ones. The
exact weight of each category of factors is still a debatable issue; however, no
human being can achieve his or her genetic growth potential under
long-lasting unfavourable nutritional and environmental conditions (for
instance, the war periods in European countries). Growth and development of
the skeleton, a very sensitive indicator of physical maturing, is also affected by
socioeconomic conditions. A somewhat haphazard, unbalanced and often
insufficient diet is one of the causes of deficiencies in both height and weight,
as are, as far as height is concerned, mother's height, birth weight and
mother's parity.[23] In contrast, the secular growth increase under favourable
circumstances illustrates the links between environment and growth, as
illustrated by the National Child Development Study in the UK[21] and the
international growth and development surveys coordinated, in eight countries, by the International Children's Centre between 1951 and 1976.[26]

One cannot speak about child development without considering psychosocial maturation and school achievements — with caution, since the debate
'nature versus nurture' is even more complex in this field, and sometimes
ideologically tinged.[27] Children of socially disadvantaged families are far too
often doomed to failure at school. However, a misleading impression is that

they seem less gifted than others from an educational viewpoint: an unskilful use of the IQ test will of course confirm this impression.

This leads to the all too frequent hasty inference that these children are endowed with inferior intellectual capacities, which in turn leads to the establishment of special classes or institutions for compensatory education which are in fact instruments of segregation and exclusion. The reality is that these children, victims of their living conditions, inadequately stimulated by their own milieu, weighed down too early in life by worries which should not be theirs, often affected by illness and therefore absent from the classroom, cannot possibly meet the requirements of a school system supposedly offering equal opportunities to all, but in fact giving priority to the elite and reproducing social inequalities. The danger consists of the subtle and tendential reasoning developed by a certain school of thought, which takes genetic differences as a starting point for analysis of intellectual inequalities. These so-called 'genetic inequalities' are used here to justify social inequalities. However, the apparent mental deficiencies of many poor children are in reality a 'pseudodeficiency' caused by social conditions. On this score, the school should be an ideal setting for exhaustive studies helping to disprove this dangerous myth, as it should also provide adequate means for the true improvement of opportunities for underprivileged children.

Given the importance of educational achievements for the future of the individual — not only for socioprofessional integration, but also for the better management of one's health — this increased risk of school failure is a heavy handicap, prevention of which is of utmost value.

Frequent illnesses and injuries

'There is considerable evidence of a marked social class gradient in some aspects of childhood ill-health',[23] especially for upper respiratory tract infections, dental decay, and sensory handicaps that are either not detected or not well looked after. Statistics are hardly needed to prove this point; doctors, nurses, social workers, medical assistants in schools, all who have occasion to examine these children, are equally struck by this chronic state of bad health and, sometimes, of bad nutritional status. More frequent and longer stays in hospital for minor ailments, with sometimes quite systematic placement in foster homes, long-term sequelae of perinatal ill events, frequent home or traffic accidents, complete the pattern of morbidity.

Mental ill-health is not as well documented. Examining the relation between low income family and child psychosocial morbidity, Lipman et al, in Canada, found it significant. A random sample of 2503 interviewed in 1983 (1076 of them re-interviewed in 1987) showed three times more psychiatric disorders — conduct or emotional disturbances, hyperactivity, social impairment — in the low income group compared to the control group. Low maternal education and family dysfunction were independent variables.[28]

The question of abuse in underprivileged families must be treated cautiously. In the early surveys, child abuse was found to be more prevalent in these families, and emphasis was put on the correlation with poverty and socioeconomic difficulties. Then, many authors agreed on its occurrence in all social classes, with more social and judicial actions being taken against the poor and the well-to-do families better protecting their intimacy. With the universal increase of difficult living conditions, several recent surveys (see ref. 29 for review) again draw attention to the impact of poverty on parent–child relationships: poverty does not lead inevitably to abuse, but it increases vulnerability.

Mortality

We have already mentioned the higher risk of perinatal death for babies of poor families. For instance, 'in 1984, the perinatal mortality rate for social classes 4 and 5 in the United Kingdom was 12.2‰ compared with 7.7‰ for social classes 1 and 2'.[23] Progress benefits all classes, but unequally, and the social gradient, although progressively reduced, is still important; in France, the difference between the infant mortality rate of children of unskilled workers and that of managers' children was 2.6 in 1969 and 1.8 in 1983.[16] More recent figures will be available soon.

Access to care

'Since thirty years, a lot of surveys are reaching the same conclusions: whatever the country, the sex, the age group, the race, the disease, the poor are more ill and die earlier than the rich. Likewise, one can see that poor people, relatively to their needs, do not use health services as others'.[30] This paradoxical situation, universally acknowledged, is at the same time a failure of and a challenge for health professionals. It starts with prenatal care, with potentially harmful consequences for both the mother and her offspring; the first antenatal visit is often delayed and the number of visits is less than what is recommended locally, less than for the average pregnant woman, in spite of financial incentives and/or high-risk pregnancy. Both the British perinatal survey and the French survey 'Naître en France' have fully demonstrated this.[21,31] In the same way, antenatal technology (e.g. ultrasonography) is used more by women of higher social class and less by those of lower class, who are nevertheless more often in need of prenatal care. According to a French health economics survey, the medical consumption of children under 16 is higher if the parents are totally reimbursed (by social security and complementary insurance), if the number of children is 3 or less, and if the social milieu is high; poor families resort more to the hospitals, often for neglected symptoms or acute diseases.[32]

How can it best be understood that those more in need are those seeking less? The current trend is towards a multifactorial explanation, combining the structural approach of the Black Report:[33] financial barriers, living conditions, social organization, and the cultural aspect, which emphasizes the perceptions and representations of health and disease by the poor, the cultural distance between them and health professionals, the way (unfriendly?) in which services are delivered to the poor and to marginal people. Indeed, individual, social and environmental factors intervene, living conditions and individual behaviour are closely related to the social context. However theoretical this discussion appears, it is crucial for the necessary improvement, for rapprochement between potential users and providers.

Unfit for the future

The picture would not be comprehensive without a final broader view, taking into account other areas in addition to health. Poor health is only one of the various disadvantages — already mentioned by Robbins[20] — that potentiate each other and threaten the future of the poor, and this vicious circle must be broken in several points if the situation is to be improved.

'GOOD HEALTH IS A GOAL IN ITSELF'

This is a statement of the worldwide 1993 report of the World Bank, 'Investing in health'.[34] However, such an investment requires a broad mobilization of several factors, and the five points of the Ottawa Charter for Health Promotion provide a good framework for such an enlargement.[35] In addition, the technical discussions of the 47th World Health Assembly (May 1994) were devoted to 'Community action for health', for which one of us was the general rapporteur; we shall also use some material coming from these rich discussions.[36]

Develop personal skills

'The poor are the only experts on poverty' (Wresinski). However, this expertise is seldom acknowledged, and even less used. The basis of the 'Wresinski approach'[37] is to help this expertise emerge and to build on it. In so doing, those who work with the poor contribute to develop their resilience, their capacity to bounce back from the difficulties in their lives.[38] This area should be explored in depth, and not enough research is devoted to those individuals and/or families who cope with serious problems and risky situations in which many others would be destabilized and sometimes destroyed. The ethical value of such an approach, also largely used in Belgium, France and Quebec, for example, is clear: it restores the dignity of the poor and their self-confidence.[4] However, much support is needed, and one must be careful not to be too demanding all at once, with the risk of putting them in a situation of failure. It is unfair to say, 'You are responsible of your health', without providing the necessary skills and resources for them to exert this responsibility.[4,39]

Creating supportive environments

To start with, it is crucial not to destroy or undermine the existing networks in the community (self-help, informal groups. . .); on the contrary, they must be carefully identified, acknowledged and empowered. Any kind of social support is important and can make a difference; several examples, such as the one reported by Bouchard in Montreal[40] concerning child abuse, are convincing. Many associations and non-governmental organizations are at work in the field; they must be helped, strengthened and used, provided they work with and not for or instead of the people. The support may sometimes take the form of financial incentives or re-allocation of resources; however, providing resources without social and moral support can be detrimental and create a mentality of dependence and passiveness.

Strengthen community action

Community action for health must be understood as a global and sustainable process by which any community — either social, geographic or professional — is involved as a full partner at all stages of the health care process, from the identification of needs, selection of priorities, planning, implementation and evaluation of activities in close cooperation with the formal health sector as well as with other sectors concerned. Community action for health is at the same time a basic concept and an essential part of public health programme development. However, no community is a homogeneous body; it consists of several groups with various needs and resources and community action for health is only effective in promoting equity in health if the needs of the minorities and most disadvantaged groups are taken care of.[36] According to the Ottawa Charter, strengthening community action requires enabling people (listening to them, increasing their skills, making them self-confident), mediating and advocating. The development of personal skills and the strengthening of community action must not ignore the intermediary level, the family itself. Nothing can be done on behalf of children if the family is side-lined, and professional involvement is useless if it does not involve the family. Development of parental skills and helping the family to cope with its difficulties is the best way of protecting children and to avoid what is the main fear of Fourth World people: to be separated from their children.

Re-orientate the health service

This is perhaps the most difficult task and has at least two aspects — structural and operational — linked by a common approach, combining confidence, cooperation, support, delegation of tasks and means. Professionals have grown used to living with the comfortable idea that the increasing complexity of medical knowledge and technology make it unavoidable that they make decisions for patients. As a result, too little attention, if any, has gone to the wealth of knowledge which can be found in each and every community. Thus, the gap has widened between health professionals, on the one hand, who are expected to have the knowledge, and therefore the power to make decisions for others, and the lay public, on the other hand, who, for lack of knowledge, are supposed merely to defer to the professionals' judgement and decision. Moreover, the factors that appear to contribute to the erosion of community health activities include poverty and deprivation, especially where there has been a loss of self-esteem, of self-sufficiency and a lowering of social status.[36] 'Doctors working with children should consider ways of providing an accessible and acceptable service to socially deprived families within their area and should become advocates for socially deprived children and their families'.[23] The training of medical students and of health, social and administrative personnel must be changed if they are to be expected to work in this way, empowering children, families and communities in a common endeavour towards better health. This should be done before and after graduation, with the active participation of the deprived families themselves: living in poverty, they know better than anyone what this means.

Build a healthy public policy

The attainment of a better state of health is one of the basic hopes and wishes of individuals, families and community. Any democratic policy of health insurance and social protection should support this aspiration and help in its fulfilment. Indeed, the health and social policies of the 1980s need to be modified, 'restoring per capita government expenditure on health, social services, education . . . to pre-crisis level — as well as mobilizing the efforts of the communities in early child care and self-help activities'.[10] Recognition, financing and a legal framework seem to constitute, according to the results of many initiatives, strong prerequisites for community action for sustaining health.[36] EC observatories to combat social exclusion[12] can help identify the needs of deprived people, the new pockets and groups of poverty. The active involvement of the Fourth World movement and of the National Consultative Committee on Human Rights in the preparation of a new French act to combat social exclusion is noteworthy. This reference to the Declaration of Human Rights is the pillar on which this fight must support itself. Since communities live and act at grass-root level, central authorities have to be effective in decentralizing their power, decision-making mechanisms and finances to regional and local health authorities which are closer to the concrete needs, expectations and resources of the people.[36] 'Something for everybody, more for those most in need' must be the basis of healthy public policies, as advocated by the World Health Organization (WHO) in its 'risk approach'.[41] For Central and Eastern European countries, the transition from a highly centralized health system to the market economy is a painful process, and children of poor families are seriously affected in their access to health. Safety nets should be organized, in order to avoid a further worsening of their situation.[42]

Mobilize other sectors

Although suggested by the Ottawa Charter for health promotion, this point is not put at the same level of the previous ones. In our opinion, it deserves to be highlighted as a specific goal, since intersectorality is crucial for achieving health. Sectors that need to be involved include finance, local government, education, information and media, agriculture, social welfare, defence, water and sanitation, private sector, religious sector, non-governmental organizations, etc. However, the number and variety of partners involved — varying according to the nature of the joint activity — conveys the risk of people being lost between so many participating bodies, and one of the key roles of the health sector is to act as a bridge between the community and other sectors, and also to train community members in order to empower them in this complex joint venture.[36] This is not wishful thinking, and some successful experiments clearly demonstrate the feasibility of such an approach, such as the integrated programme of perinatal services in Quebec.[43] The European Office of WHO has recently published a monograph that lists options and initiatives aiming at bringing into play 'policies and strategies to promote equity in health'.[44] Proposed measures concern action on low income, on unhealthy living and working conditions, on unemployment, on personal lifestyles and on access to health care. For 'advocacy implies not only taking up issues such as housing conditions on an individual basis but making their problems as widely known as possible. In other words, if we are to be most effective in highlighting the plight of poor children then we must be prepared to campaign on their behalf both locally and nationally'.[23] A demanding challenge ahead!

KEY POINTS FOR CLINICAL PRACTICE

- Poor children are often in poor health, with all kinds of hazards threatening their development. Taking care of them is a priority.
- Listen to their parents: they know better than anyone what living and growing up in poverty is. Their expertise is very helpful and their cooperation is absolutely necessary.
- The health of poor children is so strongly intermingled with other problems in the field of nutrition, housing, education. . . that a global approach is needed.
- The non-medical factors that interfere with the health and disease of these patients must be taken into account. However, you cannot solve everything by yourself: a multifactorial problem requires an intersectoral

approach. You must make 'their problems as widely known as possible'.[23] In so doing, you will be a real advocate for these deprived children and families.

- The training of medical students does not prepare them to work adequately with the poorest section of the population. You need to upgrade your knowledge, skills and behaviour through experience as well as by appropriate continuous education.

REFERENCES

1 Court SDM. Fit for the future. Report of the Committee on Child Health Services. London: HMSO, 1976
2 Manciaux M. La santé des enfants du Quart Monde: un constat et un défi. Rev Pediat 1979; 3 (special issue)
3 Manciaux M. Children of disadvantaged families. Exeter: Greenwood Lecture, 1980
4 Debionne FP, Manciaux M eds. Le respect de la dignité des gens, condition incontournable de l'accès à la santé pour tous. In: Le droit des familles de vivre dans la dignité. Sciences et Service: Paris, 1984: pp 1–13
5 Centre International de l'Enfance. Mouvement ATD Quart Monde. La santé des enfants et des familles du Quart Monde dans les pays industrialisés. Etude des besoins et implications pour les services, la formation et la recherche. Paris: CIE, 1985
6 Debionne FP. Pour vaincre l'exclusion de la santé, prendre les familles très défavorisées comme inspiratrices et partenaires. Cah Méd Soc 1992; 36: 303–307
7 Villermé C. Tableau de l'état physique et moral des employés dans les manufactures de coton. Paris: Edhis, 1979
8 Mansel Prothero R. People on the move. World Health 1984; 6: 11–13
9 Rosenfeld JA. Emergence from extreme poverty. Paris: Science et Service Fourth World, 1989
10 Cornia GA. Global socio-economic changes and child welfare: what will the 21st century bring us. Florence: UNICEF Innocenti Centre, 1990
11 World Health Organization. WHO in a new Europe. Copenhagen: WHO European Office, 1993
12 Commission of the European Communities. EC observatory on national policies to combat social exclusion. Athens. Institute of Educational and Vocational Guidance, 1993
13 Bradshaw J. Child poverty and deprivation in the UK. London: National Children's Bureau, 1990
14 Institut national de la statistique et des études économiques. Données sociales. Paris: INSEE, 1993
15 Institut national de la statistique et des études économiques. Les enfants de moins de 6 ans. Paris: INSEE, 1992
16 Manciaux M, Jestin C, Fritz MT, Bertrand D. Child health care policy and delivery in France. Pediatrics 1990; suppl: 1037–1043
17 Short P. Some possible principles to guide MCH policy making. Washington, DC: American Health Committee for Policy Reform, 1990
18 Colin C, Lavoie JP, Poulin C. Les personnes défavorisées. Québec. Bibliothèque Administrative, 1989
19 Wresinski J. Grande pauvreté et précarité économique et sociale. Paris. Journal Officiel de la République Française, 1987
20 Robbins D. Child in poverty. Report to the congress: children and families with special needs. Athens: 1991, pp 1–10
21 Wedge P. Born to fail? Social disadvantage — the facts and the practitioner concern. London: National Children's Bureau, 1974: pp 6–14
22 Goldstein H. The effects of maternal age, parity, social class, height, degree of preeclampsia and smoking in pregnancy on birth weight. In: Butler NR, Alberman E, eds. Perinatal problems. Edinburgh: Churchill Livingstone, 1969

23 Spencer NJ. Poverty and child health: an annotation. Child Soc 1990; 4: 352–364
24 Papiernik E. Le coefficient de risque d'accouchement prématuré (CRAP). Presse Med 1969; 77: 793–794
25 Bureau de la Statistique du Québec. Statistiques périnatales. DSC Maisonneuve-Rosemont, 1992
26 Centre International de l'Enfance. Croissance et développement de l'enfant. Publications et index 1951–1976. Paris: CIE, 1977
27 Manciaux M, Tomkiewicz S. Childhood mental deficiency. Paris: INSERM, 1983. See also the US book by C. Murray et al. The bell curve, 1994
28 Lipman EL, Offord DR, Boyle MH. Relation between economic disadvantage and psychosocial morbidity in children. Can Med Assoc J 1994; 151: 431–437
29 Straus P, Manciaux M, Gabel M, Girodet D, Mignot C, Rouyer M. L'enfant maltraité. Paris: Fleurus, 1993
30 Colin C, Ouellet F, Boyer G, Martin C. Extrême pauvreté, maternité et santé. Montréal: Saint Martin, 1992
31 Manciaux M, Rumeau-Roquette C, Fender P, Bréart G. Perinatal morbidity and mortality, an epidemiological approach. In: Stern L, Vert P. Neonatal medicine. Paris, Masson, 1987: 2–42
32 Triomphe A, Fardeau-Gautier M. Aspects économiques de la prise en charge des jeunes. In: Manciaux M, Lebovici S, Jeanneret O, Sand EA, Tomkiewicz S, eds. L'enfant et sa santé. Paris: Doin, 1987
33 Townsend P, Davidson N. Inequalities in health: the Black Report. London. Penguin Books, 1982
34 World Bank. Investing in health. World development report 1993. New York: Oxford University Press, 1993
35 World Health Organization, Health and Welfare Canada, Canadian Public Health Association. Ottawa Charter for health promotion. Ottawa, 1986
36 World Health Organization. Community action for health. Technical discussions. 47th World Health Assembly. Geneva. WHO, 1994
37 International movement ATD Fourth World. The Wresinski approach: the poorest partners in democracy. Paris: Fourth World, 1991
38 Grotberg E. Promoting resilience in children: a new approach. Birmingham: University of Alabama, 1993
39 Manciaux M, Pissarro B, Zucman E. Ethics and health promotion. Health Promot 1987; 2: 1–3
40 Bouchard C. Communication — 9th Congress of the International Society for Prevention of Child Abuse and Neglect. Montreal: ISPCAN, 1984
41 Backett EM, Davies M, Petros-Barvazian A. The risk approach in health care. Public health papers Geneva: WHO, 1984
42 Safety nets for children in Central and Eastern Europe. Summary report of a round-table discussion. Int Child Health 1991; 2 (2)
43 Colin C, Tétreault J. Le programme intégré des services prénatals globaux. Montréal: DSCExpress, 1991; 15: pp 1–3
44 Dahlgren G, Whitehead M. Policies and strategies to promote equity in health. Copenhagen. WHO Regional Office for Europe, 1993

Index